Analytical Approaches to EMS

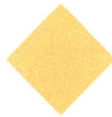

Keith A. Monosky, PhD, MPM, EMT-P

Associate Professor
Central Washington University
Ellensburg, Washington

EMS Management Series

SERIES EDITOR, *Jeffrey T. Lindsey, PhD, PM, EFO, CFO*
Distance Education Coordinator
for the Fire and Emergency Services Programs
University of Florida
Gainesville, Florida

PEARSON

Boston   Columbus   Indianapolis   New York   San Francisco   Upper Saddle River
Amsterdam   Cape Town   Dubai   London   Madrid   Milan   Munich   Paris   Montreal   Toronto
Delhi   Mexico City   São Paulo   Sydney   Hong Kong   Seoul   Singapore   Taipei   Tokyo

Publisher: Julie Levin Alexander
Publisher's Assistant: Regina Bruno
Editor-in-Chief: Marlene McHugh Pratt
Product Manager: Sladjana Repic
Program Manager: Monica Moosang
Development Editor: Kay S. Peavey, iD8-TripleSSS
Editorial Assistant: Kelly Clark
Director of Marketing: David Gesell
Executive Marketing Manager: Brian Hoehl
Marketing Specialist: Michael Sirinides

Project Management Lead: Cynthia Zonneveld
Project Manager: Julie Boddorf
Full-Service Project Manager: Munesh Kumar, Aptara®, Inc.
Editorial Media Manager: Amy Peltier
Media Project Manager: Ellen Martino
Creative Director: Jayne Conte
Cover Image: Shutterstock/B Calkins
Composition: Aptara®, Inc.
Text Font: Times Ten LT Std

Credits and acknowledgments borrowed from other sources and reproduced, with permission, in this textbook appear on the appropriate pages within text.

Library of Congress Cataloging-in-Publication Data

Monosky, Keith A.
   Analytical approaches to EMS/Keith A. Monosky, PhD, MPM, EMT-P, associate professor, Central Washington University, Ellenburg, Washington.
      pages cm. — (EMS management series)
   Includes bibliographical references.
   ISBN-13: 978-0-13-262449-7
   ISBN-10: 0-13-262449-4
   1. Emergency medical services. 2. Emergencies—Decision making. 3. Emergency management. I. Title.
   RA645.5.M66 2015
   362.18—dc23   2013023857

ScoutAutomatedPrintCode

PEARSON

ISBN 13: 978-0-13-262449-7
ISBN 10:   0-13-262449-4

Dedication

This book is dedicated to my wife, Judy, who's been my constant supporter and inspiration. She keeps me focused and motivated to do what's important to me and to the EMS profession, but keeps me grounded in what's important in life as well. Thank you for your confidence in me and never-ending love. I would also like to dedicate this work to my parents, Tony and Millie, who always had faith in me whatever it was I attempted. And, last, my gratitude and acknowledgement goes out to all of the selfless and caring EMS professionals who do what they do every day without hesitation—we are all grateful for your efforts.

—KEITH A. MONOSKY

Contents

Chapter 4

Financial Analysis   65

Chapter 5

Cost-Benefit Analysis   99

Chapter 6

Chapter 7

Chapter 8

Preface

EMS has evolved since its inception and has faced many struggles and challenges along the way. As the profession matures into an autonomous, respectable discipline, it becomes increasingly accountable to society and responsible to itself for its future direction. For this to occur effectively and efficiently, EMS practitioners must employ precise and proven analytical approaches to the profession's growth and strategic decision-making processes.

This text provides the necessary foundation for effective and adaptive analysis of EMS systems and organizations. By applying the principles and practices in this book, the EMS manager, administrator, or provider can avoid common mistakes in decision making and problem solving. In addition, the analytical approaches presented will better reveal the true nature of perceived problems through identification of the underlying causal factors and will enable identification of a more effective solution to the identified problems. The approaches can be applied in concert with one another or independently as stand-alone tools. The analytical processes can be applied sequentially or, in select cases, as needed, based upon the nature of the problems or opportunities presented to the organization.

Many of the theoretical concepts behind these analytical approaches are borrowed from other disciplines with proven effectiveness and reliability. The reader is encouraged to explore the recommendations in each chapter to expand one's scope of understanding of system and organizational analysis. The content is rich in illustration and referential details, but it is tailored for application to the discipline of EMS.

ORGANIZATION OF THIS TEXT

This text provides the reader with a foundational understanding of various analytical approaches that are applicable to EMS organizations and EMS systems. Although each chapter can stand alone in its content and instructional purpose, the average reader is encouraged to proceed through the chapters sequentially as that approach may yield the most confluent understanding of all the analytical principles in the text. This sequential approach is best for the reader who wants to become more familiar with a holistic perspective of analytical processes. By comparison, should an individual be faced with an organizational or EMS system problem that can be remedied with a specific approach, the applicable chapter can be easily examined for guidance. In this approach, the text can serve the reader well as a reference for future challenges.

Chapter 1 addresses the concept of analysis in general and its applicability to EMS. It details the essential elements of an analytical approach and why they are important. Each component of analysis is introduced so that the reader can select which component is most applicable to the challenge at hand. In addition, a brief description of the final analysis report is offered.

Chapter 2 introduces the reader to the critically important elements of problem identification: an area that is often ignored and a common source of improper analysis and problem resolution. This chapter explores innovative and effective means of ensuring proper problem identification, including mind mapping and the application of logic models.

The chapter continues to explore the theoretical concepts behind rational thinking in problem solving and how to avoid common biases and errors in judgment.

Chapter 3 constitutes a broadly encompassing foundation toward all aspects of analysis by describing fundamental principles of research. This chapter contributes greatly toward building a firm foundation of analysis by applying common research principles in the analytical approach to problem resolution. Unlike most scientific research (including medical research) that EMS providers are familiar with, this chapter introduces a somewhat different analytical foundation that has greater applicability toward organizational and system analysis. The principles and concepts in this chapter will greatly support the investigational inquiry one may have in a system or organization problem or opportunity. Chapter 3 is replete with concepts and principles that can have widespread application to the operational aspects of EMS.

Probably one of the most avoided aspects of system or organizational analysis is that of financial analysis. Most folks feel intimidated by the enormity and foreign nature of financial processes. Chapter 4 provides an easy to understand and very useful approach toward the analysis of an organization's financial picture. Common financial concepts and tools are introduced in a user-friendly manner that will enable the reader to apply effective financial analysis tools and techniques to their organization—whether they are used for problem resolution or simply to gain a clearer picture of an organization's financial performance. As important as this chapter is to the overall analytical approach, it is a very useful resource for any EMS manager as a stand-alone chapter to guide financial analysis.

Chapter 5 extends the principles of financial analysis in Chapter 4 into the familiar, but often misunderstood, concept of cost-benefit analysis. Often confused with cost-effectiveness,

cost-benefit analysis (referred to by some optimists as benefit-cost analysis) is an interpretation of some venture or acquisition relative to its social and material values. Cost-benefit analysis relies very heavily on the impacts of a decision or choice and the values it derives, both monetarily and perceptually. The very important steps and principles in cost-benefit analysis are described in this chapter with real-life EMS applications.

Closely related to cost-benefit analysis, but drawn from policy analysis, is impact analysis. Impact analysis is the subject of Chapter 6. A systematic process of impact analysis is described that helps the reader to discern the differences among varying alternatives to solutions of a problem or approaches to an opportunity. The reader will likely find many unexpected, but useful, applications of impact analysis once the concepts are mastered. Once again, real-life EMS examples are used to illustrate the utility of impact analysis.

In Chapter 7, feasibility analysis is discussed. In this analytical approach, assessing the feasibility of a choice, opportunity, or expenditure is measured beyond simply the financial considerations. In feasibility analysis, other considerations of equal importance must be contemplated and analyzed before a final decision or choice is made. Feasibility analysis may employ financial analysis, cost-benefit analysis, and even impact analysis as supportive processes, but it also considers technical and political feasibility as well.

The final chapter, Chapter 8, describes the preferred manner in which each analytical approach presented in the previous chapters should be compiled. Each analytical approach has its own strengths and weaknesses, but when combined each has a multiplied benefit to the overall outcome. When properly compiled with the findings of each analytical process, the collective results should be reported in a formal document. Chapter 8 describes the content of the final report and how it should be constructed to serve as a final determination or recommendation to stakeholders.

Analytical approaches in EMS may consist of one, several, or all of the prescribed elements contained in this text. *Analytical Approaches to EMS* can easily serve as an introductory text providing foundational instruction in each of the analytical concepts. In addition, it has been designed to serve as a useful reference for problem analysis or opportunity assessments as they arise within an organization. It is an essential tool for any EMS manager, administrator, or provider with a focus on leadership.

FEATURES

Chapter Objectives: Objectives are identified at the beginning of each chapter and outline the material the reader should understand upon completion of the chapter.

Key Terms: Key terms are listed at the beginning of each chapter and are bold upon introduction in the chapter. Each chapter's terms are defined at the end of the chapter, and all terms are included in the comprehensive glossary at the end of the book.

What Would You Do? Case Study: Every chapter starts with an EMS manager tackling some issue related to public information and education that is related to the content of the chapter. How he resolved the issue based on information in the chapter is presented in the What Would You Do? Reflection feature at the end of the chapter.

Best Practice: Every chapter includes a real-world example that illustrates information from the chapter having been used successfully by an EMS agency.

Sidebars: This feature relates interesting information that corresponds very closely to text discussion.

Review Questions: Students are required to draw on the knowledge presented in the chapter to answer the questions.

References: A list of bibliographical references appears at the end of each chapter.

ROAD MAP/HOW TO USE THIS TEXT

Anyone interested in learning how to truly identify problems in an organization or EMS system will benefit from this text. Applying the principles and concepts of analysis in this text will enable the reader to more effectively investigate problems or gauge the value of a new opportunity in EMS. The text reveals its greatest value when all chapters are applied collectively; however, for the busy EMS professional, each chapter can provide invaluable resources in its respective area of discussion. Certain chapters provide greater benefit when read first, such as reading Chapter 1 and Chapter 2 before reading any of the remaining chapters, but this is not essential. In addition, Chapter 3 provides an essential foundation for all forms of analysis and should probably always be included in the analytical approach.

TEACHING AND LEARNING PACKAGE

For information on instructor resources, including PowerPoint presentations and assessment tools, please contact your Brady sales representative.

ACKNOWLEDGEMENTS

To the wonderful people at Pearson: Marlene Pratt, Monica Moosang, and Lois Berlowitz. In particular, the editorial prowess of Kay S. Peavey in her review of the manuscript.

To Jeff Lindsey for his guidance and innovative leadership.

To all the reviewers for their incredibly valuable input and advice that helped to improve the text.

To all those who will take the time to read this text to improve EMS for the future—I thank you. Your commitment toward professional improvement and enhancement is a testimony to your dedication to the discipline of EMS.

REVIEWERS

I would like to thank the following reviewers for their feedback:

Melissa Alexander, Ed.D., NREMT-P
Instructional Designer
Greenwood, IN

David S. Becker, MA, EMT-P, EFO
EMS Program Director
Sanford-Brown College
Fenton, MO

Wally Grooms, M.Ed., NREMT-P, CCEMT-P
EMS Instructor
Central Arizona College
Chandler, Arizona

George Hettenbach, M.S.
Adjunct Professor
Delaware County Community College
Havertown, PA

Dennis Mitterer, MS, BSN, EMT-P
Board of Certified Safety Professionals
American Society of Safety Engineers
American Insurance Institute—Risk Management
Pennsylvania Nurses Association
American Nurses Association

Geoffrey L. Shapiro
Director, EMS and Operational Training
The George Washington University
Emergency Health Services Program
Washington, DC

Douglas P. Skinner, BS, NREMTP, NCEE, PI
Education Coordinator
Physicians Medical Transport
Herndon, VA

Mike Taigman, MA
Assistant Professor
University of Maryland, Baltimore County
Baltimore, MD

Michael S. Vastano, BS, AAS, NREMT-P
Training Specialist
Captain James A. Lovell Federal Health Care Center
North Chicago, IL

About the Author

KEITH A. MONOSKY, PhD, MPM, EMT-P

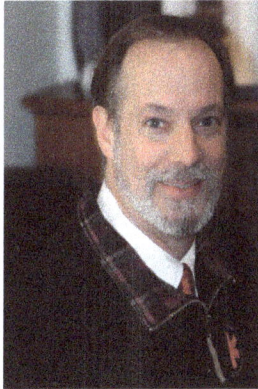

Dr. Monosky is an Associate Professor at Central Washington University (CWU) in Ellensburg, Washington, where he serves as the Director of the EMS Paramedicine Program. He has been active in EMS for more than 42 years as an EMS provider, educator, administrator, researcher, and author. He has developed numerous curricula for EMS over the years and currently administers a four-year bachelor's degree program in EMS Paramedicine at CWU.

Dr. Monosky earned his doctorate in Health Policy at The George Washington University in Washington, DC. He earned his master's degree in Public Management of Health Systems at Carnegie-Mellon University in Pittsburgh, Pennsylvania, and a bachelor's of science degree in Behavioral Neuroscience at the University of Pittsburgh.

He previously held positions as the Program Director for the graduate program in Emergency Services Management at The George Washington University, where he was an Assistant Professor in the Department of Emergency Medicine. He has also served as the Director of Operations for a large for-profit EMS agency, an EMS Specialist for the University of Pittsburgh Medical Center, a Research Coordinator for the University of Pittsburgh, an Instructor for the Center for Emergency Medicine in Pittsburgh, and the Director of EMS for the McKeesport Hospital EMS System.

Dr. Monosky currently is a Commissioner for the Commission on Accreditation of Allied Health Education Programs, a member of the National Association of EMS Educators (NAEMSE), a member of the National Association of EMS Physicians (NAEMSP), a member of the Wilderness Medical Society, a guidelines committee member of the Committee on Tactical Emergency Casualty Care (C-TECC), and an active member in the Kittitas County Search and Rescue team. He and his wife, Judy, enjoy hiking and backcountry camping with their two dogs in the Cascade Mountains.

About the Series Editor

JEFFREY T. LINDSEY, PhD, PM, EFO, CFO

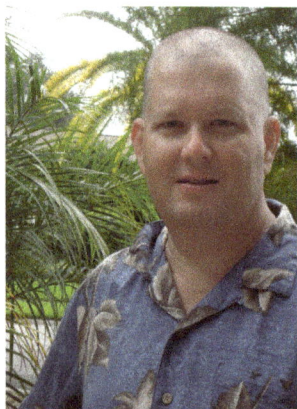

Dr. Jeffrey Lindsey has served in a variety of roles in the fire and EMS arena for the past 30 years. He has held positions of firefighter, paramedic, dispatcher, educator, coordinator, deputy chief, and chief. He started his career in Carlisle, Pennsylvania, as a volunteer firefighter/EMT. In 1985 Dr. Lindsey pioneered the first advanced life support service in Cumberland County, Pennsylvania. He is retired as the Fire/EMS Chief for Estero Fire Rescue, where he served as the South Division Incident Commander during major events. He was also part of the Area Command for Lee County EOC. Currently he is the Distance Education Coordinator for the Fire and Emergency Services Programs at the University of Florida.

He has served as an inaugural member on the National EMS Advisory Council, representing fire-based EMS, and is a past member of the State of Florida EMS Advisory Council, where he served as the firefighter/paramedic representative. He currently serves as representative to the Fire and Emergency Services Higher Education EMS degree committee. He has been active in the IAFC, serving as liaison to ACEP and attending various meetings representing fire-based EMS, and as the inaugural chair of the Community Paramedic committee, and he is an associate member of the Prehospital Research Forum.

He was a monthly columnist on product reviews for 3 years for The Journal of Emergency Medical Services (JEMS), a national EMS journal. He is a columnist for Firerehab. com and has authored numerous fire and EMS texts for Brady/Pearson. He is currently the Chief Learning Officer for the Health and Safety Institute, which produces 24-7 EMS and 24-7 Fire videos. He also was an EMS professor for St. Petersburg College (Florida).

Dr. Lindsey has been involved in a number of large events and has served within the incident command system at the upper level, including during a number of wildland fires and Hurricane Charley. He has also been involved in the preparations for a number of other hurricanes and tropical storms.

He holds an associate's degree in paramedicine from Harrisburg Area Community College, a bachelor's degree in Fire and Safety from the University of Cincinnati, a master's degree in Instructional Technology from the University of South Florida, and a Ph.D. in Instructional Technology/Adult Education from the University of South Florida.

In addition, Dr. Lindsey has completed the Executive Fire Officer Program at the National Fire Academy. He has designed and developed various courses in fire and EMS. Dr. Lindsey is accredited with the Chief Fire Officer Designation. He also is a certified Fire Officer II, Fire Instructor III, and paramedic in the state of Florida; holds a paramedic certificate for the state of Pennsylvania; and is a certified instructor in these and a variety of other courses.

Dr. Lindsey has an innate interest in alternative health. He is a certified nutritional counselor, a master herbalist, and a holistic health practitioner.

About FESHE

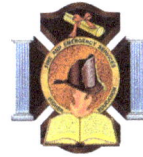

FESHE (Fire and Emergency Services Higher Education) is a dedicated group of individuals from around the country. It is hosted by the United States Fire Administration through the National Fire Academy. The mission of this group is to develop a uniform model curriculum for associate's, bachelor's, and master's degrees. In December 2006, a group of EMS educators convened as the inaugural EMS committee for FESHE. The mission was to develop a model curriculum in EMS management at the bachelor's level. It was the consensus of the leaders across the United States that the committee focus on the management issues of EMS. The clinical portion of the industry is addressed through the National EMS Education Standards and is mainly focused at the associate's level.

This text is written to meet the needs of the national model curriculum for EMS management at the bachelor's level. The EMS management curriculum includes six core courses and seven elective courses. Following are titles in Brady's *EMS Management Series,* designed to meet the FESHE curriculum.

CORE

- Foundations of EMS Systems
- Management of EMS
- EMS Community Risk Reduction
- EMS Quality Management and Research
- Legal, Political and Regulatory Environment in EMS
- EMS Safety and Risk Management

ELECTIVE

- Management of Ambulance Services
- Foundations for the Practice of EMS Education
- EMS Special Operations
- EMS Public Information and Community Relations
- EMS Communications and Information Technology
- EMS Finance
- Analytical Approaches to EMS

What Are Analytical Approaches and Why Are They Necessary?

Objectives

After reading this chapter, the student should be able to:

1.1 Describe the historical perspectives of EMS that make problem identification and resolution difficult.

1.2 Demonstrate an understanding of why analysis of an organization or EMS system may be necessary.

1.3 Identify common circumstances that make an effective analytical approach in EMS essential.

1.4 Describe the components that constitute the analytical approach.

Key Terms

analytical design

cost-benefit analysis

evidence-based
  practice

feasibility analysis

financial analysis

impact analysis

integrated analytical
  report

problem identification

SWOT analysis

WHAT WOULD YOU DO?

The Board of Commissioners for your county has approached your organization's leadership and asked for a report on whether or not EMS services should be expanded to neighboring communities due to the recent collapse of the surrounding EMS systems (Figure 1.1). There are many considerations in this potential endeavor. Does your organization have the necessary resources? How much expansion would be necessary? How many staff would need to be hired? Can your organization and the county afford this expansion? What will be the impact of the expansion to the existing service communities? What are the likely political consequences? What factors caused the collapse of the preexisting EMS system? These are just a sample of the questions that you may need to consider. How will you address this request, and what aspects need to be examined for you to render an informative response?

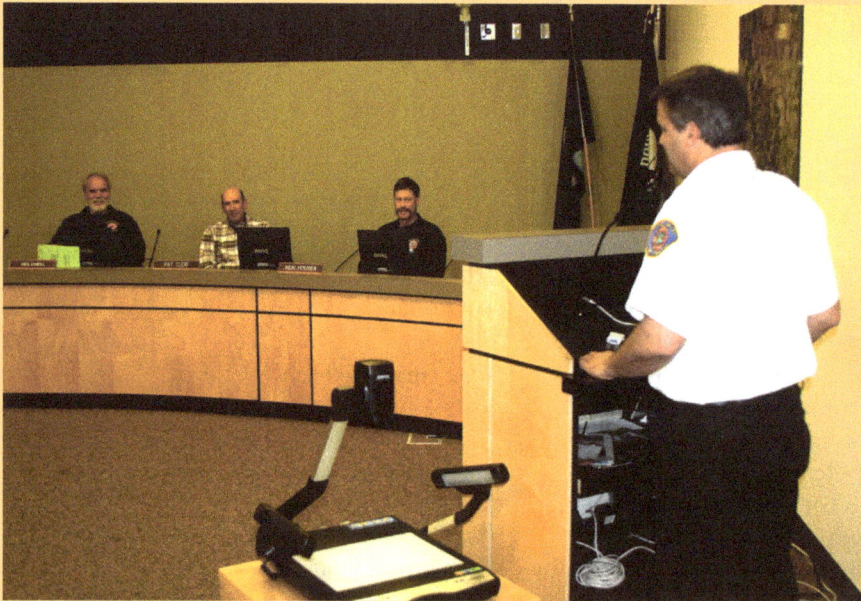

FIGURE 1.1 ■ The County Commissioners present a request to investigate expansion.

■ INTRODUCTION

Many would consider emergency medical services (EMS) to be a young profession, establishing its formal existence by most accounts in the mid-1960s (Division of Medical Services, 1996). Despite its recent inception, EMS has undergone considerable change and growth. Much of the development was well directed and purposeful, but unfortunately some of it was a product of instinct, opinion, and even unsupported beliefs. Without a central guiding force, EMS evolved in a somewhat disjointed fashion throughout various regions of the United States. This fragmented growth pattern is evidenced by the wide differences in the organizational models—such as for profit, not for profit, municipal based, fire based, etc.—that developed to meet local needs and the variances in the delivery models of emergency prehospital care across the United States—such as tiered response, first response only, etc. (National Highway Traffic Safety Administration, 2008). The diversity of EMS in the United States is further evidenced by the fact that common organizational types and structures of EMS delivery systems tend to be somewhat more prominent in differing geographic areas (Federal Interagency Committee for Emergency Medical Services, 2011). Some regions of the United States have more municipal agencies, more private organizations, or more fire-based organizations than others. Figures 1.2, 1.3, and 1.4 illustrate the geographic variances associated with differing EMS agency types.

Source: "2011 National EMS Assessment" Federal Interagency Committee for EMS, National Highway Traffic Safety Administration.

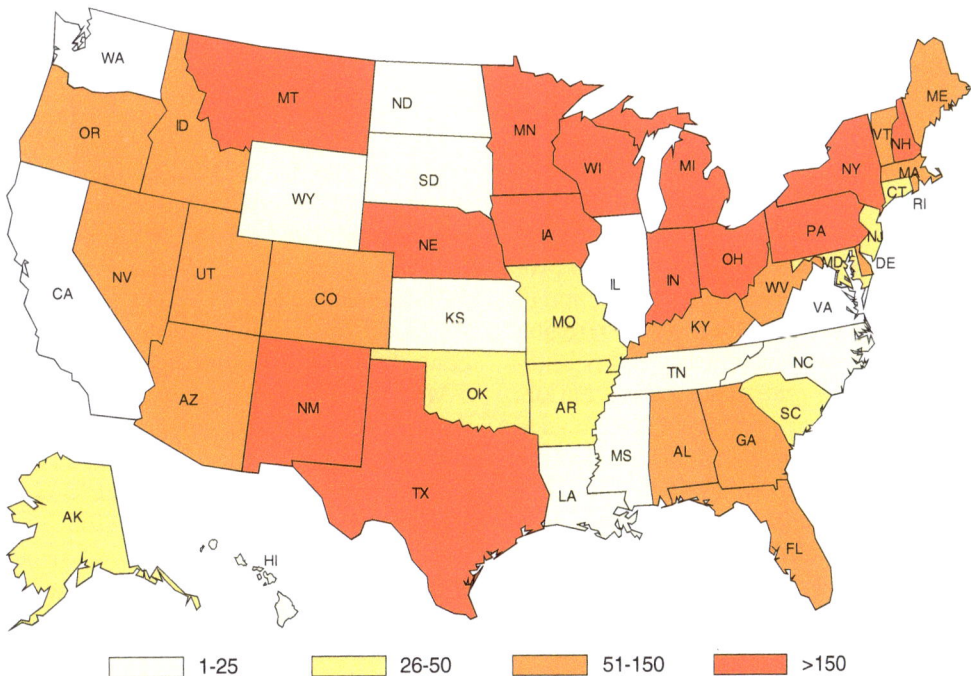

FIGURE 1.2 ■ Fire-based EMS agencies in the United States. *Source: National Highway Traffic Safety Administration, 2011.*

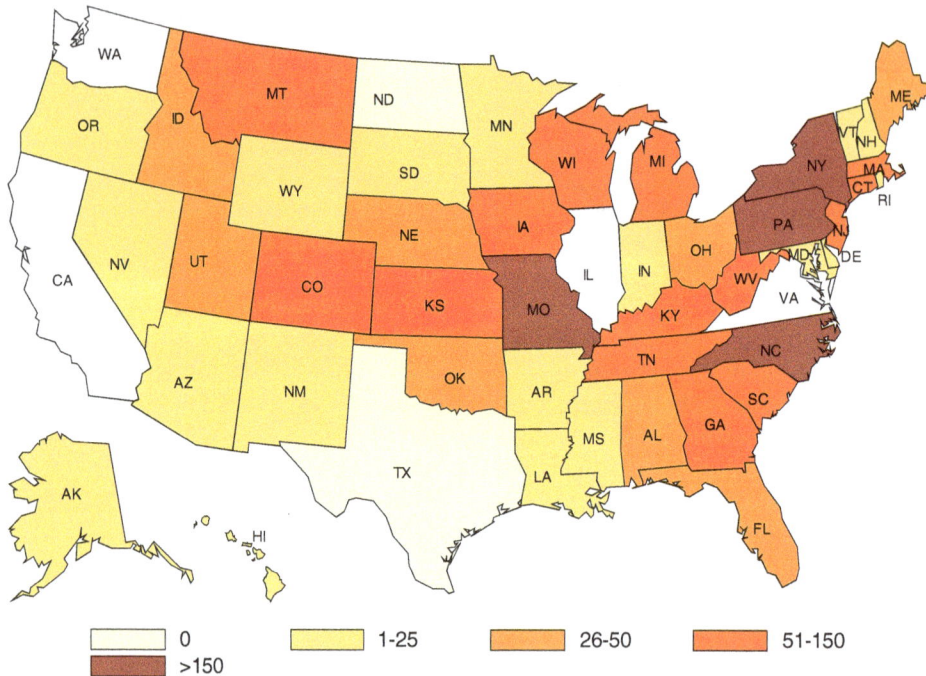

FIGURE 1.3 Governmental, Non-fire-based EMS agencies in the United States. *Source: National Highway Traffic Safety Administration, 2011.*

In addition, and perhaps more important, the delivery of emergency care and medical practices are also nonstandard throughout various geographic locations. The treatment protocols, interventional methods, or utilization of medical devices vary considerably from region to region. Some areas routinely employ interventions such as rapid sequence intubation, the administration of prehospital fibrinolytics, the routine application of capnography, or the innovative use of ultrasonography in EMS, whereas others do not. These examples help illustrate the non-uniform nature of EMS in the United States. The 2007 IOM Report, *EMS at the Crossroads,* clearly cited the fragmented nature of EMS nationwide and its apparent separation from the overall health care system in the United States as being problematic (Institute of Medicine, 2007). More recent

investigations have revealed the stark variances in scope of practice interventions between rural and urban EMS systems as well as EMS agency types (Williams, Valderrama, Bolton, et al., 2012).

As a fairly young profession lacking a central guiding force throughout its evolution, EMS has developed into a varied collection of isolated initiatives intended to provide effective emergency medical care based on anecdotal experiences. What is lacking is an evidentiary basis for change or directed growth. This has become a recent concern as **evidence-based practice** is influencing the operation and delivery of EMS nationwide. Sometimes, empirical evidence guides us away from how we've always practiced. To accept new approaches, we must maintain an open mind.

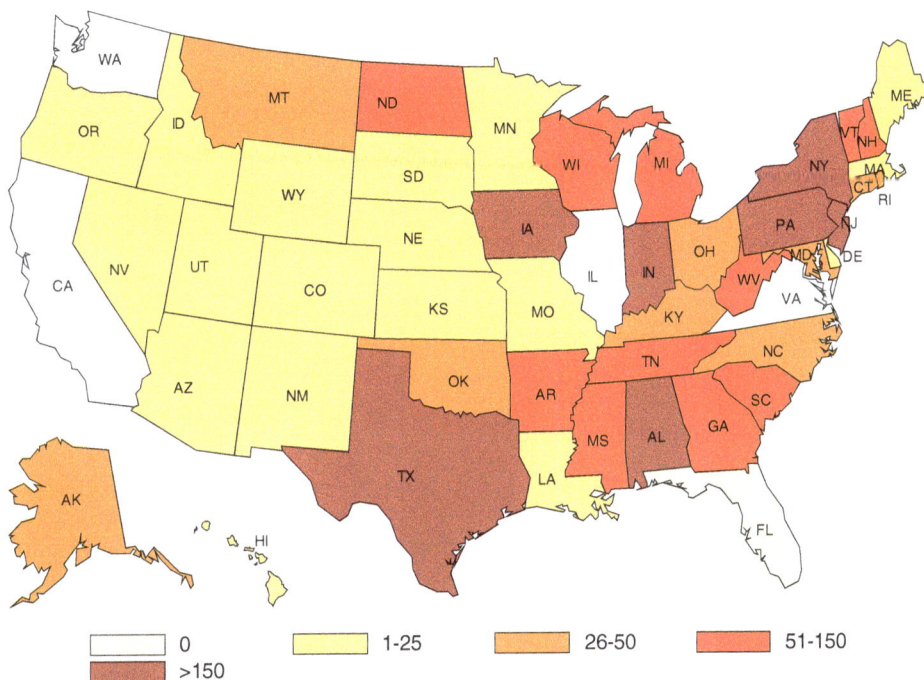

FIGURE 1.4 ◼ Private, non-fire-based EMS agencies in the United States. *Source: National Highway Traffic Safety Administration, 2011.*

◼ WHY IS AN ANALYTICAL APPROACH NECESSARY?

Diversity creates challenges that are sometimes difficult to identify and often difficult to resolve. The aforementioned variances among and within EMS delivery systems nationwide make problem identification and problem resolution particularly difficult to remedy. To effect change and work toward standardization nationwide, a reliable and consistent means of **problem identification** is needed, a process that clearly exposes weaknesses and deficiencies within an EMS system, proposes a generalized and concerted effort toward evidence-based practice and operation, and provides an effective method of achieving problem resolution and national policy changes that benefit EMS.

Many well-intentioned EMS leaders have expended significant effort to correct some of the problems and shortcomings inherent in EMS in the past. How can one tell if these efforts were effective or directed at the actual source of the problem—and, for that matter, if the source was accurately identified? These have been some of the many challenges facing EMS, and certainly they can be attributed to being products of a fragmented system.

One means of gauging progress, avoiding known mistakes, and identifying potential problems is to compare EMS to other professions. Fortunately, some parallel professions and proven concepts can help EMS focus future growth and avoid spurious or ineffective changes. To effectively apply these borrowed corrective measures, EMS leaders must consider what problems (or opportunities) exist within EMS systems and how to quantify those identified problems, develop solutions to those problems, measure the effectiveness of applied solutions, and determine, in advance, the likely impacts those solutions may have on the system.

As mentioned, a growing amount of attention is being paid to evidence-based medicine, particularly in the interventional practices and care delivered to patients. That same emphasis needs to be applied to the assessment of the EMS system, or to any of its components. By correctly identifying system problems, developing solutions that are effective, and preliminarily predicting their impacts, we can ensure that the EMS systems can grow and develop with the greatest level of success and support.

The need for correctly identifying problems, potential challenges, and opportunities for development in EMS is considerable. In the past, many EMS managers would respond to circumstances and organize a rapid solution to challenges as best they could with what minimal tools were available. Today, we can borrow proven analytical approaches from other disciplines, tailor them to the purposes of EMS, and apply them effectively to render better outcomes and less waste of resources.

As the profession of EMS continues to grow and becomes an integral part of the overall health care system, the importance of performing effective analysis and implementing appropriate and cost-effective changes becomes increasingly essential. It is also apparent that recognizing significant problems in EMS and rendering appropriate solutions will likely be subject to greater public scrutiny as EMS becomes an increasingly relevant component in overall health care. For these reasons, we must arm ourselves with the tools and the talents necessary to identify issues, draw reliable conclusions from unbiased data, and generate alternative solutions that satisfy the majority, if not all, of the stakeholders in

EMS. This approach represents a somewhat new venture for most EMS leaders and decision makers, so a structured and detailed process is important.

■ WHY IS ANALYSIS IMPORTANT?—

To help illustrate common applications, as well as the importance of an analytical approach to EMS, consider the following scenarios:

Scenario 1: Your quality improvement manager has reported that evidence suggests the paramedic staff is having difficulty clinically differentiating patients with respiratory difficulties secondary to pulmonary edema to that of pneumonia. You are interested in quantifying the magnitude of those differences and what approach would be most effective in correcting the problem while maintaining minimum cost.

Scenario 2: Your local board of commissioners has indicated its desire for you to expand your EMS services into a neighboring community. This would almost double your service demands. Is this a feasible option? How many EMS staff and support personnel would you need to hire? What would be the total cost to the organization for this expansion? What alternative solutions exist for this expansion, and how well will the commissioners accept your recommendation?

Scenario 3: Your agency provides only primary EMS and fire response to your community and currently contracts with a third party to provide EMS transport. Another, independent provider has expressed interest in serving as the principal transport agency. Its proposal is attractive, but will it meet the needs of your agency and the community? What is the financial solvency of the new organization? How does it compare to the existing contracted agency?

Scenario 4: You are contemplating adding another ambulance to your fleet. How much can you afford to spend on a new unit? Will it meet the growing demands for your service? What would be the best way to finance the purchase of this unit? What is the financial life of this unit? Will this purchase be cost effective to the community?

Scenario 5: Personnel in your organization have been asking management to acquire an optically guided endotracheal intubation device to improve intubation performances. You have been hesitant because of the cost. In the past, management has abided by the personnel's requests but has occasionally found its recommendations to be a bit biased and unfounded. How can you avoid the mistakes of past practices and use reliable evidence to support your decision?

EMS leaders face these, and many other similar scenarios, every day. The situations are often resolved by what is believed to be proper utilization of available resources, seemingly correct advice from outside interests, and an overall impression of what might be best for the organization with, unfortunately, little empirical evidence to support it. Each of these scenarios could be better informed by a proper analysis of the situation. The tools and concepts to accomplish these analyses are provided in the chapters that follow.

This text intends to provide readers with an understanding and means of effectively analyzing problems or growth opportunities within their EMS system. Problems and opportunities come in many forms and from many sources; the principles in this text are adaptable to most situations and will likely prove to be useful in many instances. To accomplish those goals, EMS leaders must

have an arsenal of analytical approaches to match the variety of situations that they may face. For that reason, each chapter will focus on one, important aspect of analysis. Even though each chapter can stand alone to provide instructional details in the analysis of an EMS problem or the evaluation of a prospective opportunity, the reader is strongly encouraged to consider every chapter in order to build their full scope of understanding and skills in analysis and to be prepared for any situation that may arise.

COMPONENTS OF ANALYSIS

This text focuses on the most common, applicable, and productive of approaches. It is essential that one become familiar with all components of analysis to ensure a thorough process. Some components complement each other, whereas others serve to fill a purpose that no other components can satisfy. In addition, some components are foundational to the analytical process and should be incorporated with each analytical attempt.

PROBLEM IDENTIFICATION

Analysis generally always begins with either a presenting opportunity or problem identification—a concept that is familiar to most of us—but efforts along these lines arc often misguided. Problems are frequently based in what is believed to be true or what was identified as problematic in the past. Although it is human nature to fall victim to what is familiar, or what is instinctually correct, we've come to appreciate in medicine that the best approaches to care are not always what is perceived to be best choices—and so was born evidence-based medicine. This valued approach can be applied with great benefit to other problems or issues within EMS. The best methods for closely examining situations and identifying the nature of actual problems must be learned.

It cannot be emphasized enough that problem identification is a crucial step. If the perceived problem is not correctly identified, then all of our analytical efforts will be futile and our corrective resolution ineffective. Proper problem identification is foundational to the analytical process, regardless of our analytical approach.

ANALYTICAL DESIGN

Once the problem has been properly identified, we can begin building our analytical approach by establishing a firm foundation through the development of a proper **analytical design**. This is best accomplished with a thorough understanding of the elemental principles of research design. To accomplish this, one must examine the different types of research, the benefits and shortcomings of the various types, which designs are best suited for particular problems or opportunities, and how to go about designing the ideal research model for analysis.

Research models may vary by design or type, depending on the most suitable approach to the problem. Whether they are quantitative, qualitative, or both in design, they remain an objective means of analysis. It is important to recognize that research endeavors can have many different forms—each form having specific advantages and disadvantages in application. In medicine, for example, many consider the double-blinded, randomized, clinical trial of quantitative research as the gold standard. This is merely one form of research that has a particular utility for clinical research. It does not have utility in the discovery and potential resolution of many EMS system problems. For that reason, an analyst must be familiar with other forms of research and be willing to apply them appropriately.

Once the research model has been decided upon, it should be supported with theoretical

concepts, and an understanding of some real-life examples, as well as a review of common resources to aid in research development. An excellent resource example is the National EMS Information System (NEMSIS)—a developing system for national EMS data compilation. From this level of development, one can explore how to build a detailed analysis using this important foundation and ensure it progresses in the direction appropriate to serve the identified problem or opportunity.

Side Bar

National EMS Information System (NEMSIS)

Funded by the Centers for Disease Control and Prevention (CDC) and the National Highway and Transportation Safety Administration (NHTSA), NEMSIS emerged from the standards set forth by the "Emergency Medical Services Agenda for the Future." It was formed in 2001 under the direction of the National Association of EMS Officials and the guidance of Greg Mears, M.D.

NEMSIS represents a national effort to collect and compile EMS data into a single, accessible repository of useful prehospital information. Through the evolutionary development of its data-set standards (currently employing version 3), the organization has enabled a compilation of information that has great value to researchers, educators, administrators, and any others with interest in health care trends, health measures, and demographics.

One benefit with incredible potential is the provision of real-time surveillance through a process known as syndromic surveillance where a constellation of symptoms is recognized early for potential onsets of epidemics, instead of waiting for diagnoses or lab values. This approach gives public health officials an early warning of outbreaks of illness or the emergence of unusual injury patterns.

Once the foundation of the analysis has been established through the development of the research design, continued analysis can then proceed in several different directions to achieve the necessary focus. Often, this next phase will encompass multiple components. Each optional component at this stage of analysis must be fully understood so that the appropriate analytical processes can be selected for application to our identified problem or opportunity. Any one of these optional components may prove to be necessary or useful in your final analysis. For that reason, it is important to understand the applicability and limitations of each component and appreciate its utility in the overall analytical process.

FINANCIAL ANALYSIS

Although not essential for the analysis of every problem, there are a few circumstances in which **financial analysis** is not expected or does not become invaluable. In many situations, this component is often the most important, but frequently it is the least often applied of all analytical processes—often because it seems so foreign to us or too difficult to apply. For financial analysis to be effective, one must understand the many concepts and tools of the financial analytical component and how they can be applied to many problems or opportunities.

Financial analysis is often not applied because of its intimidating nature for many people. However, you needn't be a CPA or financial guru to figure out some of the basic economic problems or financial warning signs that may be embedded in your EMS system or organization. Simply looking in the right places and with some degree of insight and understanding of the basic analytical tools of finance will make the problems quite apparent.

FEASIBILITY ANALYSIS

Another important consideration is the realm of **feasibility analysis**. This is usually applied to a particular business or investment venture. Often compared to a **SWOT analysis**, a feasibility analysis is a general assessment of the benefits and consequences of considering a business venture, such as expanding services, initiating a new program, or acquiring new equipment. A SWOT analysis determines an organization's strengths, weaknesses, opportunities, and environmental threats. Although feasibility analysis (or SWOT analysis) is a popular concept, it has inherent limitations, as it often relies on subjective assessments and interpretations. To be effective and contributory to an analytical approach in EMS, feasibility studies must be based on objective findings and empirical data. This can best be accomplished if feasibility analyses are enhanced with other components of analysis.

COST-BENEFIT ANALYSIS

The next component to consider is an important analytical approach that has gained increasing value among federal agencies in recent years: **cost-benefit analysis**. Cost-benefit analysis (CBA) is different from cost-effectiveness analysis, a common misunderstanding among most who entertain applying a CBA. There are many subtle and important differences between a CBA and a cost-effectiveness analysis. A core difference is the consideration of the societal value of alternatives in a CBA. In effect, a CBA determines if the endeavor is worth doing. Therefore, a thorough understanding of the basic elements in conducting a CBA is essential to any effective analytical approach. Most major ventures in any organization that involve significant allocation of resources—whether it be operational growth, acquisition of expensive equipment, expanding the scope of services, or even changing an organization's mission or vision—should probably be accompanied by a cost-benefit analysis.

IMPACT ANALYSIS

Once all of the necessary information has been obtained in the initial phases of analysis, deciding on the most appropriate and effective solution or course of action depends on assessing the impact of the preferred approach and comparing it to that of alternative approaches. To effectively conduct analysis in an organization or EMS system, one must always consider conducting an **impact analysis**, a critical aspect of decision making in EMS. Impact analysis can be applied to policy decisions or in situations where client or political preferences should be taken into consideration. Often, impact analyses center around specific goals that are evaluated by predetermined impact categories. This way, alternatives can be more effectively compared in terms of impacts and outcomes. As such, impact analysis provides a unique value to the analytical process and, therefore, should accompany every form of analysis in EMS.

INTEGRATED ANALYSIS REPORT

To complete the analytical process, one must consider the integration of each of the aforementioned analytical components into a final product in order to generate a cogent, detailed, and final **integrated analytical report**. The end user or benefactor of the analytical approach must be able to glean considerable detail, perspective, and reliable information from the analysis report in order to make the best decision. The information and details in the integrated analytical report, which is a formal document, should be fully supported and findings should be appropriately referenced when necessary. Often, these analytical reports offer alternative solutions with one or several recommendations for the decision maker to consider. Rarely are they conclusive in nature. Having a clear understanding of the elements and proper format of the analytical report is critical to the entire analytical process.

CHAPTER REVIEW

Summary

In review, once the problem or opportunity for organizational growth has been properly identified, a strategy for applying the analysis should be made and the chosen analytical components employed. With the information gained from the analytical approaches, the data are compiled to inform a preferred decision or course of action, and alternatives are formulated as well. This entire process is summarized in a final integrated analytical report for consideration by the organization's leadership.

The general principles of organizational and system analysis, as well as each of the aforementioned components, form a foundation for EMS leaders and decision makers to effectively conduct meaningful analyses of their organization or EMS system. Although most useful during periods of crisis, the emergence of a problem, or unanticipated opportunities of growth or expansion, these analytical approaches may be used otherwise to inform EMS leaders or decision makers so they may acquire a clearer understanding or insight into the nature of the challenges they may be facing. Once the reader is familiar with the components of analysis, this text would serve well as a reference for the future. The sources listed in the References section at the end of this chapter will help in learning more about the many aspects of EMS system analysis.

WHAT WOULD YOU DO? Reflection

First, you must recognize that this is an opportunity for growth. Putting the challenge facing you into writing will help to define the task: "Is it feasible for our existing EMS organization to expand its coverage into neighboring communities? What are the benefits, what are the risks, and what are the consequences?"

Next, you would begin to identify growth opportunities by diagramming possible processes though a mind map or logic model. You would also want to research similar challenges to other EMS organizations. Your analytical process should begin with designing the proper research methods in order to discern the information that you'll need. Consider the financial implications, the cost versus benefit values, the feasibility of the existing organization to handle such a sizable increase in capacity, and the impact that the expansion and any alternatives may have on all involved stakeholders. Finally, you will integrate what you learn from your varied analytical approaches and incorporate that into a condensed and informative report for the commissioners to consider.

Review Questions

1. Why does the profession of emergency medical services have uniquely significant challenges in problem identification and resolution?
2. What is regarded as the first, and perhaps most important, step in EMS system analysis?
3. Which step is considered to be foundational in all other components of analysis?
4. What specifics are essential in considering the necessary analytical design in EMS system analysis?
5. Why is financial analysis so important in the analytical approach?
6. What is a fundamental difference between cost-effective analysis and cost-benefit analysis?
7. What is another name for feasibility analysis?
8. What does an impact analysis consider?
9. What qualities or characteristics should an analytical report include?
10. How does learning the various analytical approaches help an EMS leader?

References

Division of Medical Services, Committee on Trauma and Committee on Shock. (1996). "Accidental Death and Disability: The Neglected Disease of Modern Society." Washington, DC: National Academy of Sciences-National Research Council.

National Highway Traffic Safety Administration. (2008). "Configurations of EMS Systems: A Pilot Study." Washington, DC: U.S. Department of Transportation.

Federal Interagency Committee for Emergency Medical Services, National Highway Traffic Safety Administration. (2011). "National EMS Assessment." Washington, DC: U.S. Department of Transportation.

Institute of Medicine, Committee on the Future of Emergency Care in the United States Health System. (2007). "Emergency Medical Services: At the Crossroads." Washington, DC: National Academies Press.

Williams, I., A. L. Valderrama, P. Bolton, et al. (2012). "Factors Associated with Emergency Medical Services Scope of Practice for Acute Cardiovascular Events." *Prehospital Emergency Care* (16)2, 189–197.

Key Terms

analytical design The basic structure of the analytical approach, based on general principles of research. The analytical design is variable and dependent on circumstances and informational needs.

cost-benefit analysis An analytical process, financially based, that compares the aggregate net benefits of an endeavor with its aggregate net expenses.

evidence-based practice Conducting an activity that has reliable, empirical evidence to support its implementation.

feasibility analysis An analytical process that helps to determine if an endeavor can be implemented given the nature of the organization, the mission of the organization, and the operational environment; often compared to a SWOT analysis.

financial analysis A process of analysis that involves a close examination of financial performances, usually through organizational financial statements and financial ratios.

impact analysis A process that examines the potential impacts of various goals and compares those outcomes among differing alternatives; also known as policy analysis.

integrated analytical report The final report of the analytical approach. It is concise, detailed, informative, and well referenced. Minimally, it consists of an introduction, background, problem identification, analytical design description, data collection methods, results and interpretations, alternative solutions, and recommendations.

problem identification The initial step in the analytical process; it ensures the correct identification of a problem or opportunity through a variety of analyses.

SWOT analysis A common strategic planning approach that examines the strengths, weaknesses, opportunities, and threats of an organization; often compared to a feasibility analysis.

Problem Identification

2 CHAPTER

Objectives

After reading this chapter, the student should be able to:

2.1 Describe the complexity of problem identification and its importance, including the need for multiple revisions and the value of empirical information.

2.2 Recognize that biases and preconceived notions may erroneously influence problem identification.

2.3 Describe the general, overall approach to problem identification and commonly applied approaches.

2.4 Describe the process of mind mapping and the application of logic models in problem identification.

2.5 Describe the importance and application of conducting literature searches on the identified problem.

2.6 Explain bounded rationality and how it applies to problem identification, problem solving, and decision making.

2.7 Identify common biases and errors in judgment, and describe how to avoid them in problem identification processes.

Key Terms

activities
agency theory
bounded rationality
confirmation biases
feedback loops
informational
   asymmetry

inputs
literature search
logic model
mind mapping
outcomes
outputs
root cause analysis

selection biases
self-serving biases
subjective expected
   utility

13

You are the director of a midsize EMS agency serving an urban–suburban municipality of approximately 200,000 residents over approximately 90 square miles. Your system provides a tiered-response by local fire services, as well as a contracted private EMS agency that provides only basic life support and transportation capabilities. Your agency provides both advanced life support as well as transportation capabilities. Your quality-improvement manager tells you that the paramedics are achieving only about 60 percent of the threshold for intubations on cardiac arrest patients. He asks permission to invoke a mandatory training session to improve the success rates of intubation by the agency paramedics. What should you do? Can you reliably attribute poor performance by the paramedics as the reason for the 60 percent performance rate of intubations in cardiac arrest? Are quality-improvement indicators the only measure of performance or problem resolution? Do you think your quality-improvement manager has identified the problem?

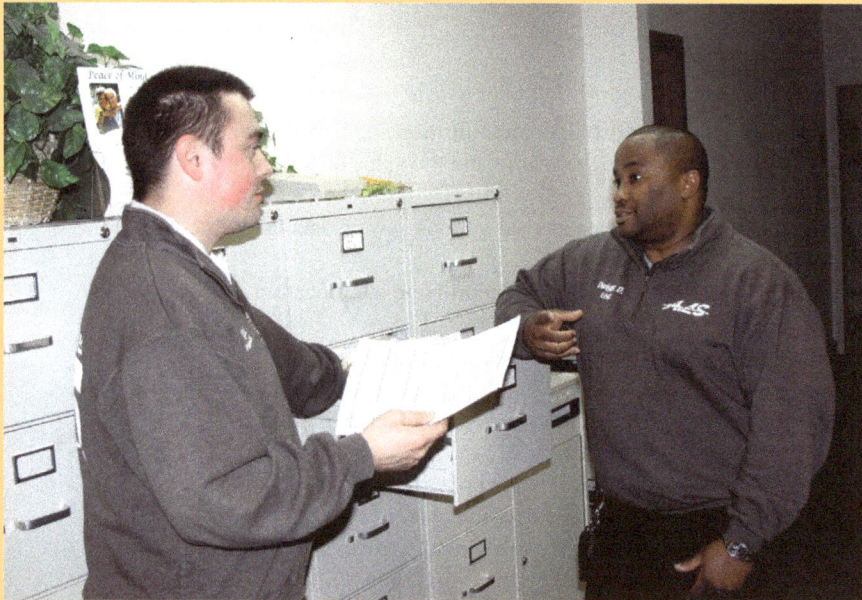

FIGURE 2.1 ■ The QI manager expresses concern regarding paramedic skill performance.

■ INTRODUCTION

Problem identification can be somewhat of a challenge despite its apparent ease. What one considers a problem may very well be a symptom of a greater underlying problem or just a perception. The challenge rests in identifying the actual problem—not simply what appears to be the problem. As most of us have experienced at some time, what once was believed to be the suspected problem actually turned out to be simply the incidental or secondary result of a greater, underlying problem. To drill down to the basis of most problems demands some degree of investigation and objective assessment. This form of investigative approach will be explored in this chapter.

A few introductory cautions are necessary. First, it is essential to avoid trying to identify the problem in terms of the solution. This is one of the most common sources of incorrect problem identification—most people tend to confuse problems with solutions. How many times have you heard one of the following? "The problem with this system is we don't have enough personnel." "Why can't management fix the problem? All it takes is a little bit of money." It is easy to assign a solution to an apparent problem, but doing so can lead the unsuspecting person down a well-worn path that often fails to actually fix the problem (because it was never truly recognized) and unnecessarily wastes considerable resources.

Second, don't rely on initial impressions of the alleged problem. Remain open-minded to actual evidence. Realize that whatever the problem may appear to be initially, it will likely be different once hard evidence is accrued. A common mistake inherent in human nature is to perceive problems based on other people's perceptions or to unknowingly employ one's own biases to the thinking process. True analytical approaches are objective, evidence based, and devoid of personal prejudices. It is

often wise to conduct some introspection of one's own view of a problem and ensure that no biases are influencing thought. Reflect on the quality of one's thinking and make it the foundation of ongoing self-assessment. This is not always easy but can be made easier with proper analytical approaches.

■ WHAT TRULY IS THE PROBLEM?

The first step in problem identification is to acknowledge that the actual problem may not be what it appears to be. It is important not to be misled by appearances, general opinion, past experiences, or gut feelings. To avoid this, several things must occur.

First, approach each problem with an open mind and be willing to accept what the data offer. This requires gathering some objective (bias-free) information. Therefore, problem identification usually involves data collection and analysis—even in the beginning stages. For this reason, we must be willing to revise our initially identified problem as more information is gained. Based on new information revealed during data collection and analysis, we may discover the true nature of the problem, which may be different from what was initially suspected. So, in this initial stage, problem identification is only provisionally proposed.

In general, most analysts approach a situation with the understanding that multiple revisions of the problem may be necessary before we are confident that the true underlying problem has been identified. One of the more common obstacles in problem identification, other than not using objective findings, is an unwillingness to revise what was initially believed to be the case. Being resistant to change during problem identification will lead us down the wrong path and will result in incorrect findings and a misguided resolution. Although it is human nature to rely on emotions, past experiences, and hearsay, it is our duty to base decisions on facts—which is not always an easy task. One method to break down the perception and emotion barriers is suggested in the "Brainstorming" sidebar.

Side Bar

Brain-storming

When faced with challenges of provincial thought or close-mindedness among decision makers, consider a brainstorming session whereby rules and restrictions are abandoned and free thought is encouraged.

Set up rules that any possible idea or proposal is not off the table and innovation is welcomed. With ample encouragement, ideas begin to flow and barriers to creativity are lowered.

Be sure to assign a scribe to record the ideas on a whiteboard as they are proposed. When done, have the participants select their favorite ideas through a voting process (nominal grouping).

Nominal grouping is accomplished by having participants vote for their top three choices among the recorded ideas, and the results are then tallied.

Second, we must seek information on our provisionally identified problem from multiple sources, such as surveying different individuals on their perceptions of the problem and examining different elements of the problem. For example, if we've preliminarily identified the problem to be prolonged out-of-service times at the hospital, we'll need to interview the crews, hospital staff, and perhaps even dispatch personnel. In addition, we may need to examine out-of-service times for the different hospitals, different crews, types of calls, and what activities were necessary to put the unit back into service. This example suggests the varied nature of information collection that may be necessary to develop an objective perspective on problem identification. However, in many instances, problems of little ambiguity may emerge and, therefore, would not require such an intense level of investigation.

Third, to avoid being misled, employ as many approaches as necessary to elucidate the reality. Examining a problem with a single approach is analogous to identifying an acute myocardial infarction (AMI) with a single, bipolar limb lead. When time permits, every problem deserves a multidirectional approach toward identification. This same principle of multidimensionality will apply to our comprehensive analysis. The more perspectives or views we consider, the greater confidence we can have in identifying the problem and analyzing it effectively. This will ultimately lead to a more reliable solution. A most evident example of this principle is the concept of triangulation, whereby multiple sources of information help to elucidate a single issue or problem. Obviously, some problems are time sensitive and demand an immediate analysis. Recognize that circumstances which demand an immediate, singular analytical approach may result in erroneous results if a multidimensional approach cannot be taken due to the nature of the problem.

Even in paramedicine, when our patients are facing a life-threatening situation that demands an immediate response, we are contemplating multiple alternatives and considering differential diagnoses when deciding on an interventional course of action. To allow tunnel vision to guide our analysis limits our opportunity for the best corrective action.

APPROACHES TO PROBLEM IDENTIFICATION

Although many methods attempt to identify problems, it is important that they be systematic, inclusive, thorough, and repeatable to establish reliability. A diverse, yet comprehensive, approach is proposed here that employs mind mapping, logic models, and literature searches. These approaches are fairly standardized and have wide applicability to most problems.

MIND MAPPING

Approaches to problem identification can take many forms. When taking an open-minded and multidimensional approach to initial problem identification, one popular method is to view the problem from a more global, rather than focused, perspective. This approach is akin to mind mapping. In fact, mind mapping can easily be applied to problem identification. In general, **mind mapping** involves identifying a central theme and then brainstorming associated elements or inputs of that theme, and illustrating those relationships in a radial or interconnected fashion (Buzan and Buzan, 2010; Mindmapping.com, n.d.). Mind mapping helps tremendously in conceptualizing problems and demystifying complex challenges. Figure 2.2 illustrates a mind map of the previous example.

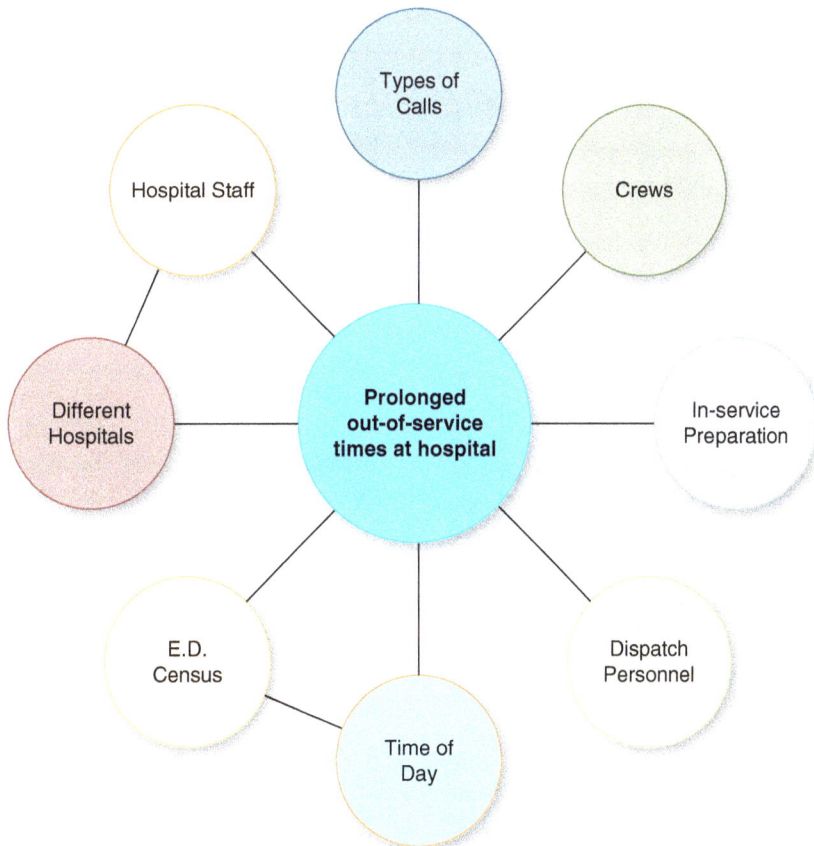

FIGURE 2.2 ■ A simple example of a mind-mapping problem.

The benefits of mind mapping are many. It can depict multiple inputs or factors and the relationships among them, as well as illustrate subordinate influences. Mind mapping is thought to represent the natural way our minds process and envision concepts, thereby improving our understanding of the conceptual foundation of problems, consolidating multiple problems, and facilitating the development of solutions. It is theorized that by arranging the inputs, ideas, and associations in a radial fashion you are structuring them in the same way that the brain functions—in a three-dimensional manner, not a linear one. In addition, using colors to represent ideas and associations enhances conceptualization as they recruit the visual functional capacities of the brain, helping to categorize associations and aiding in remembering ideas. Many resources on mind mapping are available, both in print and on the Internet. Some of these resources are listed at the end of this chapter.

LOGIC MODELS

Another important and very useful approach to problem identification is developing a logic model. A **logic model** is a graphic representations of processes and elements within the processes that help illustrate relationships between those elements and between the processes and the products that they generate (Taylor-Powell and Henert, 2008). Put simply, it is a schematic diagram of the processes involved within a defined set of parameters. The logic model illustrates the elemental steps and outcomes.

Logic models are typically used for planning, describing, managing, communicating, or evaluating a program or concept. To be effective, logic models should be visually engaging, specific to a particular purpose, appropriate in detail and, most important, illustrated on only a single page, never two or more (Department of Health and Human Services, 2010). Logic models typically include four categories of elements: *inputs*, *activities*, *outputs*, and *outcomes*.

Inputs are resources that contribute to the entire process, such as personnel, property, equipment, and even money. All relevant inputs should be listed in the logic model.

Activities associated with the problem could be work activities, interventional treatments, or monetary disbursements. Anything that utilizes resources (inputs) to produce **outputs** (products) can be regarded as an activity. In logic models, there may be multiple activities producing several outputs, and it is useful to include all that could be relevant to the problem under consideration.

Activities are linked to particular outputs, which are typically results of the process. For example, if oxygen is an input, the administration of oxygen via a non-rebreather mask would be the activity, and an improvement in the oxygen saturation of the blood would be the output. Outputs are often easier to measure than the activities that lead to them (in this example, it could be the oxygen saturation of blood,

SpO$_2$, or the arterial blood gas values, ABGs). Many quality-improvement strategies involve output measurements, and most include some type of outcome measurement as well.

The overall result is measured in the category of outcome. An **outcome** is a snapshot of the bigger picture. Outcomes may be short term, intermediate term, or long term. In the previous example, the oxygen administration that led to improved oxygen saturation could result in the patient's overall improvement (perhaps a reduction in respiratory difficulty or tissue ischemia). In medicine, outcomes are often measured by morbidity and mortality. In our focus, we are more interested in the overall consequences of the suspected problem.

These categories are not isolated and may be hard to define at times. In a logic model, each category is often quite interdependent with other categories, and a change in one will often result in changes in all of the others. Each category has a process association between it and at least one other category, and often they influence each other in their outputs and outcomes.

A complex problem can be illustrated by deconstructing it into categorical elements and representing the relationships among the integral elements through associated processes. By doing so, it becomes increasingly evident how each component influences other components and, specifically, which components are influenced within the logic model.

To better illustrate the application of the logic model in problem identification, let's apply it to a medical problem in a very simplified fashion. Let's say that there is suspicion that crews are not adequately differentiating the various pathologies of patients with respiratory difficulty. The logic model can be applied to deconstruct the elements and processes within that problem. First, let's examine the potential inputs. Figure 2.3 lists the likely inputs to consider (there could be more than those listed).

Once each of the relevant inputs has been identified, examine what activities are

- Paramedic
- EMT
- Primary education level
- Equipment for examination
- Patient acuity
- Scene time
- Time of day
- And more...

FIGURE 2.3   Some typical inputs.

associated with the problem of failing to differentiate respiratory pathologies in patients. Figure 2.4 lists some of the activities associated with that process. Again, in actual application, it would be very important to be sure to include all activities to avoid an oversight in problems identification.

In this example, the output would be the crew's determination of the patient's underlying problem or field diagnosis. Since this is a measureable parameter, it may be obtained from the patient care reports. Examples could include suspected COPD, pulmonary edema, asthma, or pulmonary emboli. The outcome in this example could be either the patient's outcome (e.g., admission to hospital, discharged to home, died) or, for the purpose of examining the problem under investigation, it may be more useful to use the hospital diagnosis. By doing so, the problem may become more evident in the analytical process. The

- Obtaining vital signs
- Auscultation of chest
- Determination of SaO$_2$
- Percussion of chest
- Presence of tactile fremitus
- Obtaining a thorough history
- Obtaining list of medications
- And more...

FIGURE 2.4   Some typical activities.

Inputs	Activities	Outputs	Outcomes
Paramedic	Vital Signs	COPD	COPD
EMT	Auscultation	Pulmonary Edema	Pulmonary Edema
Education	Percussion	Asthma	Asthma
Equipment	Pulse Oximetry	Pulmonary Emboli	Pulmonary Emboli
Pt. Acuity	Tactile Fremitus		
Scene Time	Patient History		
Time of Day	Medications		

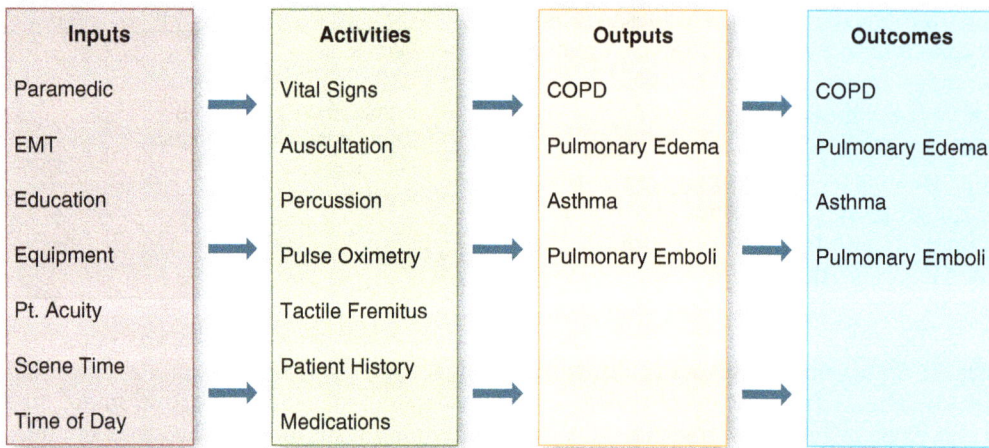

FIGURE 2.5 ■ A simple logic model—example 1.

logic model of this example is illustrated in Figure 2.5.

When examining the logic model in Figure 2.5, we can see that outputs and outcomes have the same descriptors. However, one notable difference is that one is derived by the paramedic (outputs), whereas the other (outcomes) is considered the ultimate, definitive diagnosis (from the hospital). By identifying those that are not identical, we can "work backward" to see what activities and inputs influenced those particular outputs. This would be one approach to gaining insight into the nature of the problem.

Another important component to common logic models is feedback loops. **Feedback loops** are processes or associations between elements that are used to inform or modify existing elements. For example, if a particular condition is suspected based on the patient's history and auscultation of the patient's lungs, then perhaps the paramedic may repeat a portion of the physical examination to include percussion and/or assessment for tactile fremitus. This concept of feedback is illustrated in the typical logic model as a feedback loop drawn in to denote that association.

Logic models can become quite complex. For the purposes of problem identification, it may be best to keep a logic model as elemental in scope as possible so it does not become unmanageable. It is also useful to use colors and other symbols of emphasis to help clarify relationships and associations (much like what is done in mind mapping).

Let's try one more logic model application, this time with an operational theme. Suppose your local community has leveled accusations that response times are too long. You review the past year's response times and find an average of 12 minutes for emergency responses—2 minutes over your quality-improvement threshold. What could be the cause of these delays? You can apply the logic model to help inform the problem by deconstructing the involved processes. Inputs and activities are listed in Figure 2.6 and Figure 2.7, respectively.

Once again, in this example, there may be many more inputs and activities to consider. The outputs will likely be response times, which may be categorized by time of day, geographic location, unit designation, or other limiter. The outcomes may be the performance of each category in comparison to an established threshold, such as 8 minutes or 10 minutes, depending on what the organization deems appropriate.

- Available Units
- Available Crews
- Dispatch Information
- Distances to Calls (average)
- Weather Conditions
- Traffic Conditions
- Priority of Call
- Time of day
- And more…

FIGURE 2.6 Some typical inputs.

- Dispatcher Receiving Call
- Dispatcher Dispatching Call
- Crew's Receipt of Call
- Preparation for Response
- Response to Scene
- And more…

FIGURE 2.7 Some typical activities.

By applying this approach, you can examine which outputs failed to meet the acceptable outcomes and trace back which activities and inputs may be responsible for the response delays. This will give you a general perspective of the true underlying problem. From there, you can focus your analysis by employing the components of foundational research and analytical methods, financial analysis, cost-benefit analysis, feasibility analysis, and impact analysis. A simplified version of this example's logic model is illustrated in Figure 2.8. In this illustration, the activities feed into the input to modify those elements as necessary. For example, if preparation for the call is anticipated to be long or the response to the scene is beyond a reasonable time frame, the inputs "crew" and

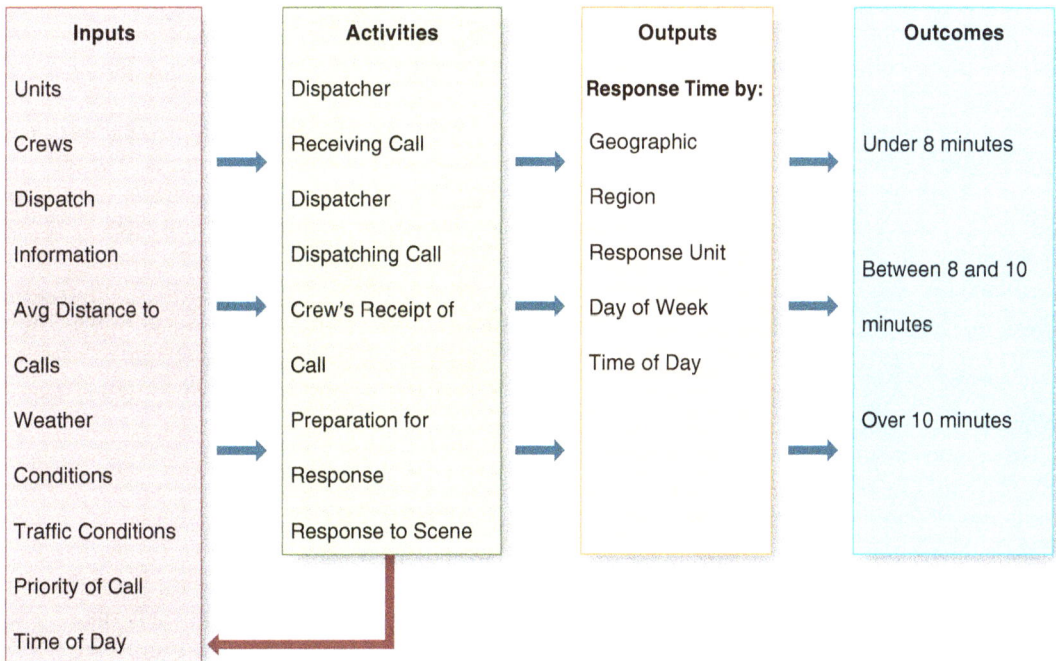

Inputs	Activities	Outputs	Outcomes
Units	Dispatcher	**Response Time by:**	Under 8 minutes
Crews	Receiving Call	Geographic	
Dispatch	Dispatcher	Region	
Information	Dispatching Call	Response Unit	Between 8 and 10 minutes
Avg Distance to	Crew's Receipt of	Day of Week	
Calls	Call	Time of Day	
Weather	Preparation for		Over 10 minutes
Conditions	Response		
Traffic Conditions	Response to Scene		
Priority of Call			
Time of Day			

FIGURE 2.8 A simple logic model—example 2.

Best Practice

The CDC Health People 2010: Objectives for Heart Disease and Stroke Prevention Programs

In 1998, the U.S Congress funded the Centers for Disease Control and Prevention to develop a series of evaluation guidelines for unifying states' approaches to the programmatic assessment of heart disease and stroke prevention activities. In response, the CDC developed a guideline for application of a logic model.

This effort not only helped to establish the *2010 Health People* objectives and national goals for heart disease and stroke, but it also provided each state's health department with a step-by-step instructional guide in the application of logic models in their evaluation efforts. This document— "State Program Evaluation Guides: Developing and Using a Logic Model"—can be found at the CDC website.

"unit" may be modified to respond additional units and personnel.

A more sophisticated logic model (illustrated at the end of this chapter), explores the processes associated with credentialing in EMS and the potential impact it might have on patient outcomes. Figure 2.10 represents a fully illustrated logic model. As you consider using logic models, you will likely find that application is easier and of greater applicability to system or operational problems. Also, the process becomes easier the more often you employ it. Try experimenting with this approach on many different applications.

LITERATURE SEARCHES

When trying to identify problems within your EMS system or organization, it may be possible that others have experienced a similar challenge. Conducting a **literature search** for identical or similar problems may be quite illuminating and informative. It may, in fact, save you a lot of time and effort if the circumstances are remarkably similar. The likelihood of finding a similar circumstance within the limited literary resources of EMS may be

somewhat remote, but it is possible that you may find in another profession a set of circumstances similar enough. System or operational problems arise often in a wide variety of professions, and identifying a similar problem in a parallel profession can be very informative to the challenge that you are currently facing.

Take the time to search the literature. You may not find identical situations or problems, but you may find some that are at least similar. There are many search engines that can provide a fairly reliable compilation of useful search results. As a general rule, when looking for literature from a professional journal, it is best to use a powerful and specific database instead of the common public search engines.

■ SOME ADDITIONAL CONSIDERATIONS

In addition to an effective approach toward problem identification, other concerns or considerations must be kept in mind when conducting such a cognitive investigation as problem identification. For one, there are limits to the human mind. Recognizing those limitations and pitfalls in cognition is an important first step in problem identification. Also, when conducting an analysis of the problem, it is usually best to employ as many analytical approaches as one can—even if you borrow them from other disciplines. Quality process assessment is a rich resource area from which we can borrow.

BOUNDED RATIONALITY

While contemplating the true nature of the problem, consider the following insights into and characteristics of human nature. It has been said that "humans are creatures of habit." We typically prefer the familiar or that which is more comfortable (in intellectual terms). Recognizing human limitations such as this helps tremendously in sorting through the minutia and arriving at a much more reliable decision. Herbert Simon, a well-respected and highly regarded social and political scientist, economist, and psychologist, helped us better understand human nature by advancing the concept of the limitations of human rationality (Simon, 1987). In his theories and writings, Simon offered several important perspectives that might prove useful in everyday efforts at problem identification and decision making:

- Problem solving and decision making are two separate activities. Problem solving is comprised of establishing agendas, setting goals, and designing actions. Decision making consists of evaluating and choosing actions. Thinking of these as separate components will help in problem identification.
- To better understand the limits of human decision making, Simon (1987) posits the theory of **subjective expected utility (SEU)**. In this theory, he proposes that all decisions are subject to maximal utility (or application) of rational thought and all relevant factors are known. In effect, this means that with each decision we make, our choices are not constrained by our

limits of rational thought and we possess all essential information necessary to make the correct decision each and every time. This approach is obviously lofty and unrealistic, but it helps us to better define our limitations in decision making.
- Central to Simon's theories, is the matter of **bounded rationality**. It is important to acknowledge that individuals are limited in their ability to arrive at perfect decisions. This is largely a product of the complexity of most situations, our limited ability to conduct intricate computations, the incomplete nature of information (**informational asymmetry**), the natural differences among people's preferences and beliefs, and the conflicts of value held by many people.

Simon (1987) recommends that we acknowledge our limits of rational thought and employ the resources available to us to render better decisions. This relies very heavily on the application of empirical research and data collection and making sure we properly frame our problem for analysis. For this reason, effective decision making and problem analysis rely very heavily on research methodology.

Simon (1987) also proposes that we must take into consideration **agency theory**, which involves the environmental setting or institutional framework in which the problem resides and in which the analysis and decision making will be conducted. (See the "Agency Theory" sidebar for more explanation.)

Side Bar

Agency Theory

Agency theory focuses on the relationship between principals (management) and agents (workforce) within the institutional environment (organization). It largely addresses conflict resolution by identifying the source and nature of the conflict.

The focus on conflict source generally centers on two typologies:

1. When desires or goals for management differ from that of the workforce
2. When the principal and agents have differing attitudes toward negative outcomes or risks

Building an organizational culture that engenders open communication and mutually agreed upon goals helps to ensure minimal principal–agent incongruence.

Another way to avoid this conflict is to ensure that both principals and agents have similar incentives for rational choices (a form of game theory) that promote congruence.

Not all problems are generalizable; that is, not every solution can "fit" every problem—all have unique properties. For these reasons, we must carefully identify our problem, frame it accordingly, and use all available resources on the nature of the problem through research and analytical processes. Only with this approach can we be assured that we've arrived at the best solution to our problem.

AVOIDING BIASES AND ERRORS IN JUDGMENT

While considering the problem at hand, we should make every effort to avoid introducing any biases that might obscure the true nature of the problem—often much easier said than done. The greatest contributor to the emergence of bias is that we often fail to recognize the conditions or circumstances that enable biases to influence our choices. When we see normal oxygen saturation readings on our pulse oximeter, should we forgo a clinical assessment to confirm the device readings? As health care professionals, we are encouraged to confirm these indicators with additional clinical evidence to avoid erroneous conclusions.

As mentioned in the chapter introduction, introspection of one's thinking processes to identify biases and ensure quality conclusions is essential. Reducing our personal perceptions is not an easy process, particularly when an emotional component is involved. When emotions play a part in any contemplation, those considerations that have emotional attachments are much more likely to rise to the surface. Separating emotional motivations from factual information is an ongoing struggle in almost all decision-making and problem-solving processes. This applies to problem identification as well.

Identifying problems that support our beliefs (**self-serving biases**) or that promote our agendas (**confirmation biases**) without evidence will likely lead us to an incorrect or ineffective solution. It is, of course, important not to allow our preferences to intrude into our consideration of potential problems (**selection biases**). Therefore, we should rely on objective measurements. Measuring the relevance, impact potential, or perceived importance of any potential problem is an important process in framing our problem. How to go about measuring these parameters involves other components of the analytical process, such as cost-benefit analysis, financial analysis, impact analysis, and causal inferences.

Errors in judgment often arise for the very same reasons. Often we make a particular choice because we are overly confident in our selection, consider it an easier choice, or simply rely on our instincts to choose the "best" problem to analyze.

One of the greatest threats to an error in judgment is informational asymmetry, in which the decision maker is not fully informed about a particular situation or problem and, as a result, an incorrect choice may be made.

Informational asymmetry creates an unbalanced situation when two parties are faced with a common problem and one party has more information than the other (which often occurs in a principal–agent relationship when one person has authority over another and uses the knowledge of information to leverage his or her position). When obtaining a medical history on a patient during assessment, should the patient fail to fully disclose vital medical information, your ability to arrive at a provisional diagnosis for treatment is severely limited. The patient is withholding information from you, creating an informational asymmetry.

Avoiding the influence of emotion and assuring oneself of full knowledge of a problem or situation will help reduce errors in judgment.

INCORPORATING PRINCIPLES OF CONTINUOUS QUALITY IMPROVEMENT IN PROBLEM IDENTIFICATION

Many principles and practices within the discipline of quality improvement have applicability in problem identification as well. Employing any of these principles can be useful if the same level of discretion and objectivity described above is maintained. Remember, no one means of analysis is foolproof or conclusive—employ as many means as is necessary to "drill down" to the nature of the problem. Also, a few words of caution in using quality-improvement tools: These methods are designed to affect change to improve outcomes on a simple issue—the problem identification process in analytical approaches is intended to identify the problem *only*, not to correct it. To achieve resolution of the problem, a more detailed and comprehensive analysis is essential. Avoid using quality-improvement tools to rectify large-scale system problems. Organizational and system

problems often have a diverse and complex nature that involve obscure causative factors for which simple quality-improvement tools cannot identify adequately.

An example of a useful and very popular continuous quality-improvement (CQI) tool is **root cause analysis (RCA)**, sometimes referred to as fish-bone diagramming because of its overall fishlike appearance in diagram form. Root cause analysis attempts to identify the actual cause of the problem, not just an exercise in sorting out and managing the consequences or symptoms of the problem. Although there are many forms and approaches to RCA, it usually consists of the following steps:

> Defining the problem—describe the problem and list all of the symptoms.
>
> Collecting data—assimilate the necessary information to illustrate the problem, its impact, and its duration of effect.
>
> Identifying the possible causes—what sequence of events led to the problem; what conditions created it; and what other problems may coexist?
>
> Identifying the root cause—this is the backbone (literally) of the RCA process. What common element or feature is found in all the symptoms and coexisting problems that can explain their existence?
>
> Deriving probability solutions—based on the analysis, what solutions would likely remedy the problem and bring about an improved outcome?

As you can see, this is a very simplified approach to analysis and, although it is useful for simple process-improvement issues, it falls short of truly identifying the actual nature of complex and comprehensive system problems. To discern these types of problems, a more varied and comprehensive analytical approach

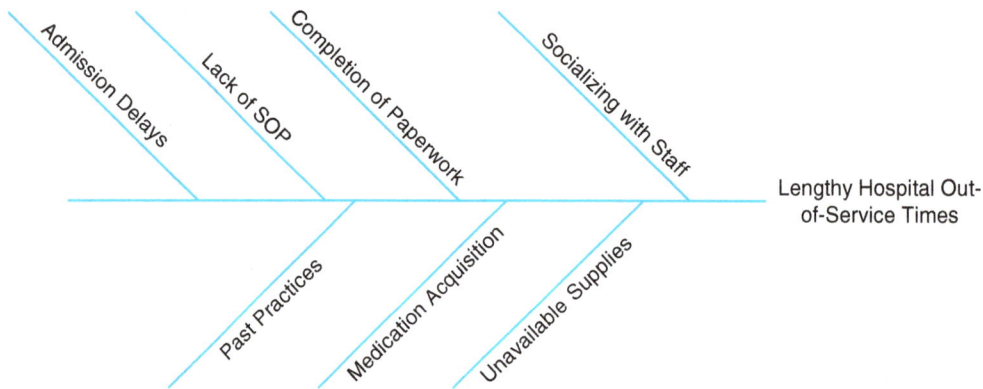

FIGURE 2.9 ■ Root cause analysis example.

is essential. Perhaps the best application of RCA in problem identification of system analysis is to list the possible contributing factors to a known problem and illustrate their interconnectivity. This application is illustrated in Figure 2.9.

CHAPTER REVIEW

Summary

Problem identification is critical to the success and outcome of the analytical processes. Although on the surface it may appear simple and fairly straightforward, problem identification may very well be complex. In addition, it is often the greatest determinant of eventual success in the analytical process. Our approach to problem identification must be open minded, without biases or emotion—in other words, purely objective and empirical in nature. We must remember that the processes associated with problem identification can also apply to defining opportunities that might present to us.

The approaches we employ can vary, depending on the nature of the problem and available resources. Nonetheless, we should familiarize ourselves with each of the means of problem identification and utilize them without hesitation. With practice, processes such as mind mapping and logic models (Figure 2.10) can be valuable, even in everyday situations. The more we apply them under routine circumstances, the more effective we become at using them in a crisis.

Problem identification involves knowing what types of problems typically exist and learning the nature of their existence. This can sometimes be best accomplished by simply reviewing the literature. Learning from others' experiences and insights is not only efficient, but it also helps us to maintain our objective approach. Similarly, recognizing our own personal limitations helps to ensure that we rely solely on objective and empirical processes in our determination of the problem. Admitting we have human limitations does not make us less human but, rather, more discerning analysts.

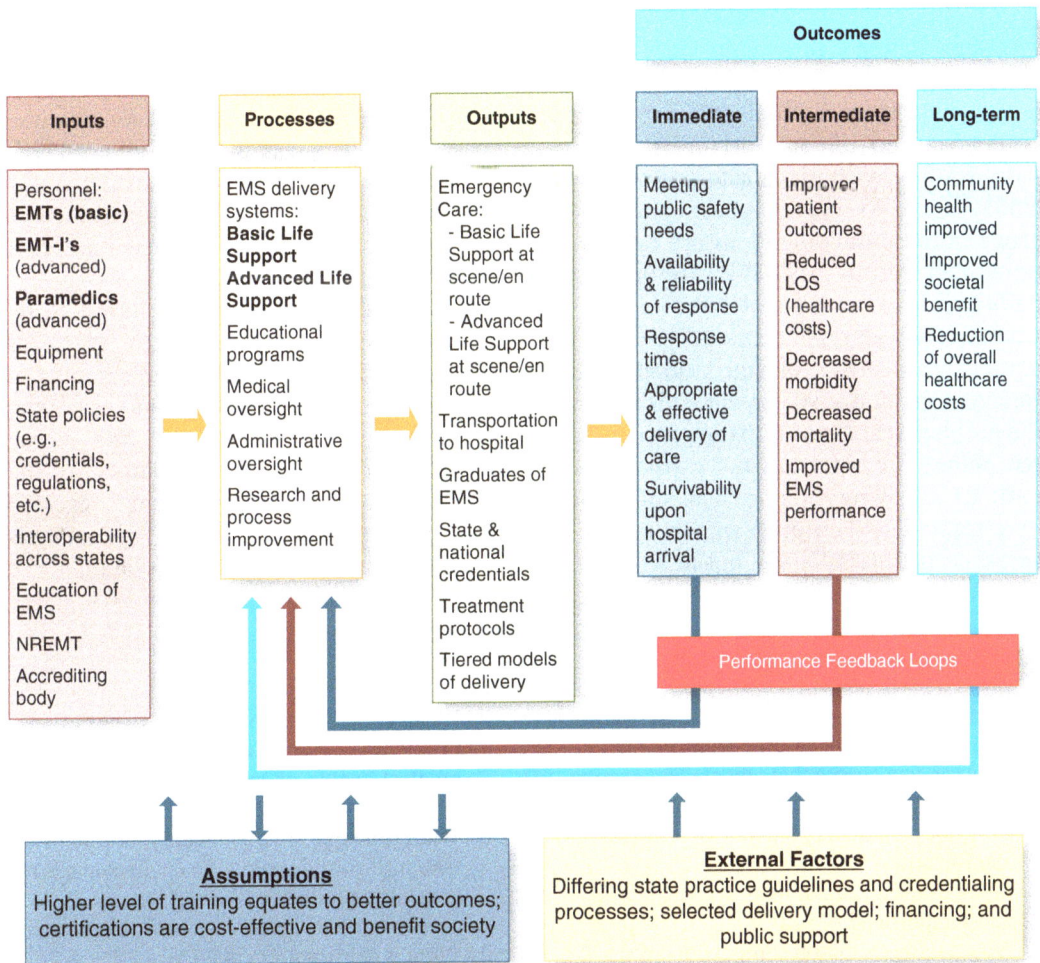

FIGURE 2.10 ■ Full-logic model of credentialing.

WHAT WOULD YOU DO? Reflection

Your quality-improvement manager has brought to your attention a potentially serious problem. Most managers and administrators would react to this information in a similar manner and authorize the implementation of a remedial education process to correct for errors in successful endotracheal intubation of cardiac arrest patients. However, being aware of the importance of identifying the true problem, you begin an analysis of the reported problem by developing both a mind map and a logic model to illustrate the elements and the processes associated with the problem. Upon doing so, you immediately identify a problem that has gone unrecognized. In peripheral coverage areas where there is a delayed response by your advanced life support units, the on-scene EMTs have initiated alternative airway management. As a result, patients in cardiac arrest in these outlying areas are being initially managed by basic life support crews before paramedics can access the patient. In situations where rapid access to patients by paramedics is satisfactory, the intubation success rates are above 90 percent. This suggests the problem is not the intubation success rate but, rather, the percentage of cardiac arrest patients receiving endotracheal intubation by paramedics. The problem, then, lies in access to peripheral areas, not in paramedic

skill performance. Identifying the problem accurately corrected the actual problem, but it also prevented a waste of resources and possible damage to staff morale.

Because you addressed the perceived problem with an analytical approach, you were able to identify the actual nature of the problem and avoid unnecessary interventions and an ineffective resolution. Relying on one, isolated approach (such as quality-improvement indicators) can lead to erroneous conclusions. In this case, the quality-improvement manager was basing his interpretation on only one aspect of the problem: quality indicators that suggested poor paramedic performance. Your analysis revealed another underlying problem.

Review Questions

1. What are some common obstacles in identifying the true nature of a problem?
2. How can you ensure that you are considering all viable explanations to a perceived problem?
3. How does mind mapping help in problem identification?
4. When drawing a mind map, why are colors often important?
5. What are the common components of a typical logic model?
6. When compared to other approaches to problem identification, what might be the greatest benefit of employing logic models?
7. What is bounded rationality?
8. What principle are you employing when you take into consideration the circumstances in which the problem arose and the organizational culture that bred the problem?
9. What is confirmation bias?

References

Buzan, T., and B. Buzan. (2010). *The Mind Map Book: Unlock Your Creativity, Boost Your Memory, Change Your Life.* Upper Saddle River, NJ: Pearson.

Mind Mapping.com. (See the organization website.)

Taylor-Powell, E., and E. Henert. (2008). "Developing a Logic Model: Teaching and Training Guide." Madison: University of Wisconsin-Extension, Cooperative Extension, Program Development and Evaluation. (See the organization website.)

Department of Health and Human Services, Centers for Disease Control and Prevention (2010) Evaluation Guide: Developing and Using a Logic Model. CDC Division for Heart Disease and Stroke Prevention. (See the organization website.)

Simon, H. A. (September–"October 1987). "Decision Making and Problem Solving," *Interfaces 17*(5), The Institute of Management Sciences, Carnegie-Mellon University, Pittsburgh, Pennsylvania.

Key Terms

activities The second level of a logic model that associates processes of inputs to achieve outputs.

agency theory The environmental setting or institutional framework in which the problem resides and in which the analysis and decision making will be conducted.

bounded rationality The limitations of human thought that prevents full resolution of problems due to their complexity, the incomplete nature of information, the natural differences among people's preferences and beliefs, and the conflicts of value held by many people.

confirmation biases Making choices based on the influences of a personal agenda.

feedback loops Informational inputs into the processes of a logic model from resultant events. Feedback loops can occur anywhere in the logic model to inform an earlier process or activity.

informational asymmetry A circumstance whereby one party has more or better information than another party and uses that information to his or her advantage; often found when one entity has authority over another, as in the principal-agent relationship

inputs The first level of a logic model that lists the resources and constituent components to the process.

literature searches Careful examinations of the current and past professionally published documents that can inform a situation or problem. These are often conducted through a professional search engine or database.

logic model A conceptual illustration that demonstrates the elemental components to a complex process to render a relational understanding and an association among those components.

mind mapping A conceptual application that illustrates relationships and associations to various elements within a common theme. The process includes a colorful depiction of components and a branching hierarchy of ideas and concepts.

outcomes The eventual result of the entire process in a logic model. Outcomes may be short term, intermediate term, or long term.

outputs The third level of a logic model that is the product of the activities applied to the inputs (or resources) in a process. They are often measureable and often short lived.

root cause analysis A tool commonly used in continuous quality-improvement practices to illustrate contributing factors to a common problem and to aid in developing a solution.

selection bias Making choices with any form of influence that is not objective but is subject to human behavioral persuasion.

self-serving bias Making a choice that provides oneself with a greater utility, despite the fact that the choice is unfounded or not factual.

subjective expected utility A theory that proposes that all decisions are subject to maximal utility of rational thought and all relevant factors are known.

Applying the Principles of Research

CHAPTER **3**

Objectives

After reading this chapter, the student should be able to:

3.1 Relate the importance of problem identification and the empirical process in the analysis of EMS problems.

3.2 Describe the various typologies of design in research, their varied purposes, and how each applies to analytical approaches in EMS.

3.3 Describe the fundamental features, common forms, differing utility, and theoretical differences between quantitative, qualitative, and mixed methods analytical approaches.

3.4 Describe the fundamental features, differences, utilities, and proper applications between descriptive, exploratory, and explanatory styles of research designs.

3.5 Describe the differences and applicability of the scientific method and the social investigative research method in analysis of EMS.

3.6 Describe the differences and applicability of experimental design approaches and that of quasi-experimental design approaches in the analysis of EMS systems.

3.7 Identify the differences and applicability of the idiographic and nomothetic forms of explanatory research in EMS analysis.

3.8 Describe the features of variables, the criteria for variable selection, units of analysis, and the operationalization methodologies for study variables.

3.9 Describe the inductive approach and deductive approach as theoretical foundations of research inquiry.

3.10 Identify the common essential considerations for executing a comprehensive research endeavor for analytical purposes in EMS.

3.11 Relate the identified problem to each of the integrative steps in the formulation of research design.

3.12 Describe the data collection process, its relevance to the research design, and its importance to valid and reliable outcomes.

3.13 Describe the different forms of validity and identify each of the common threats to internal and external validity.

3.14 Describe content analysis, its constituent types, its utility, and the common methods of application.

Key Terms

attrition effects
causality
coding
cohort study
concurrent research
confounding effects
content analysis
continuous variable
correlation
data collection instrument
deductive approach
dependent variable
empirical process

experimental design
experimenter bias
external validity
focus group interviews
Hawthorne effect
history effects
idiographic explanation
independent variable
inductive approach
institutional review board (IRB)
internal validity
key research question

latent content
Likert scale
manifest content
maturation effects
mixed methods design
nomothetic explanation
nonspuriousness
operationalization
panel study
prospective research
qualitative design
quantitative design

quasi-experimental design
retrospective research
secondary research question
selection bias
self-reporting bias
telephonic survey
testing effects
time order
trend study
typology
units of analysis
variables

WHAT WOULD YOU DO?

You manage a medium-size municipal EMS agency in an industrial-based city that has undergone some recent economic downturns. Your service has been exemplary for many years, but population growth has strained your capacity and your performance thresh-

olds are suffering. You have made the plea to the city council to add two more units and employ eight more full-time EMS providers to meet current demands. The council members have cited a significant shortfall in the budget and ask if this expansion will generate enough revenue to support itself in the first year. The city also recently laid off two police officers, and the public is outraged.

1. How should you proceed?
2. How can you go about demonstrating to the council members that your plan will be profitable? And will it?

3. How do you assess the public's sentiment about expanding the EMS force when the police force was just reduced?
4. What would be your first step?

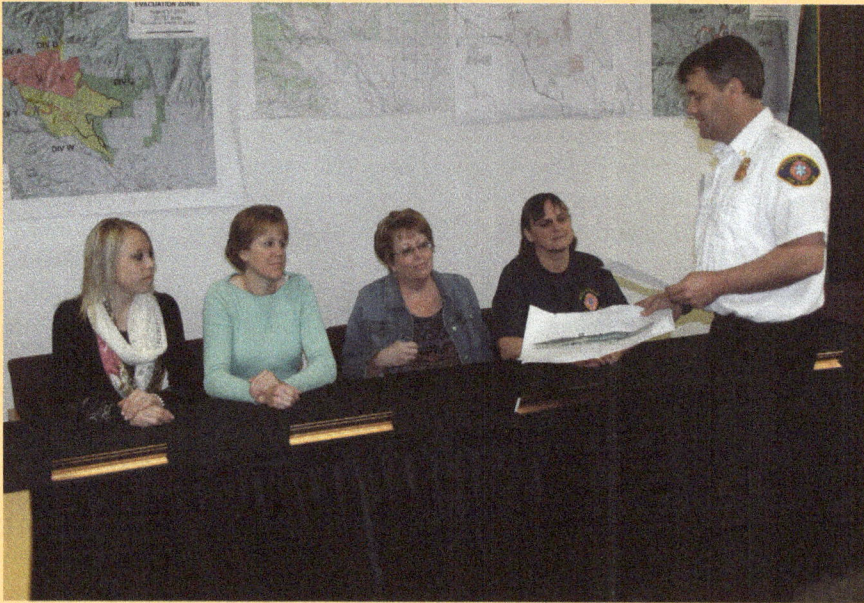

FIGURE 3.1 ■ The EMS manager pleads his case to the city council.

■ INTRODUCTION

When confronted with an unidentified problem or significant issue, we often respond initially by saying "Let's get some information to see what the problem is" or "Let's try and figure out how this came to be." In essence, it is intuitive to know that arriving at a solution necessitates knowing the details underlying the problem.

We routinely gather data when faced with a challenge so that we may get to the root of the problem. However, to ensure an effective and appropriate solution, we must gather as much of the data as is necessary to render the correct conclusion and do so methodically so as not to allow ourselves to be misled. The objective should be to gain an understanding sufficient enough to illuminate the problem clearly and avoid arriving at partial truths. Whereas it may be impossible to gather all of the available information under some circumstances, avoid the temptation to gather evidence that is abundant or apparent without delving deeply enough into the nature of the problem.

So, in this formal analysis, the process begins by accurately and reliably identifying the problem. Once the problem has been correctly identified, the data collection and analytical processes begin. Of all the analytical approaches and tools, no one technique or analytical process is more relevant and instrumental to the overall effort of problem resolution than the application of general research principles. This chapter will explore the fundamentals of how research can provide the essential analysis for most problems or opportunities presented to us. It is important to note that this chapter does not replace a formal course or textbook in research principles, but it does provide an effective overview and summary of those principles that would be most germane to system analysis for EMS.

To begin, a new approach must be taken in gathering the necessary information to learn about our problem or opportunity. No longer can we rely on instinct, hearsay, or the informed opinion of others. We must methodically collect our information in a regimented and standardized manner. It is only with this approach that we can be sure we are gathering the correct information and analyzing it properly to arrive at the best possible solution. Henceforth, we can refer to this detail-oriented process as an **empirical process**. An empirical process is one that employs a scientific method, usually through observation or experimentation. Although we may rarely conduct experiments to gather data in our effort to resolve problems, we should always collect data in a rigid and precise manner, much like true experimental processes. For this reason, we will become somewhat more familiar with standard research methodologies in this chapter.

One additional detail worthy of mention is that we are often inclined to either forgo the regimented process of data collection and analysis or we may abbreviate or lessen our efforts in these processes. It is human nature to take the easier route—whether it be traveling to work or searching for the truth. The dividends to be gained from a systematic and methodical approach far exceed what we could gain otherwise. For this reason, we should always strive to

Best Practices

Research Forum in EMS at UCLA

The Prehospital Care Research Forum at UCLA has been the driving force behind EMS research for a number of years. The forum promotes the research efforts of members of the EMS discipline, enables dissemination and recognition of research endeavors, and provides lectures and workshops for those interested in learning research methods for EMS.

The concept that the future development and growth of EMS rest with its providers is acknowledged by the Research Forum: "The Prehospital Care Research Forum at UCLA believes that it is the responsibility of emergency medical professionals worldwide to build a body of evidence to examine prehospital emergency care" represents part of the mission of the forum. Each year, research abstracts are presented at various EMS conferences though these efforts. Please visit the organization's website.

apply as many of the principles discussed in this chapter as we can in our formal analysis of a problem or opportunity.

On the other hand, research should always have a purpose, and researchers should be loyal to that purpose. We should never conduct research for research's sake, but we should strive to keep discovering new information and inform our existing collection of knowledge. Once we attain that goal, we can then revisit the need to conduct additional research.

TYPES OF RESEARCH

To better understand research methods, let's begin with examining the various ways that research can be categorized. Categorizing research methods is often helpful in determining which approach we should take for a particular problem. If we think of the nature of the category, we can better apply the correct form of research to our problem by matching the underlying **typology** of the research to the nature of our problem. The more familiar we are with the various research methods, the more likely we will be to choose the best method to arrive at the correct answers. In general, the manner in which research can be categorized is often based on design, purpose, method, and time dimension. We will explore each of these as a means of categorization.

DESIGN

Under this category, we will generalize how we intend to gather data and to analyze that data. Our initial approach here is going to be broad, but we should narrow our design type as we contemplate our problem and the methods of analysis more closely. From a very broad approach, we can consider conducting research in a quantitative manner, a qualita-tive manner, or perhaps both. Each has its own qualities, benefits, and limitations. Let's first consider a quantitative design.

Quantitative Design

In **quantitative design**, the data collected are of a numerical nature (Remember: *quant*ity is of a number of items, thus *quant*itative is numerical in nature). This may be what most people think of when they think of research—the traditional scientist who is conducting experiments in his laboratory and recording measurements (in numbers) of each event that takes place. Quantitative research has been around a long time and researchers are quite familiar with these methods and the relevance of their results. In fact, our level of understanding of quantitative research has led us to believe that this approach is the most evident and revealing of the underlying cause of many events. Scientists often refer to quantitative research as the most "robust" of research. However, robust (like many descriptors) depends on one's perspective. In recent years, social scientists have demonstrated that other methods of research may be equally robust—a subject that we will also discuss in this chapter.

It may be apparent that to conduct quantitative research, one must collect numbers as some means of measurement. This interpretation is entirely true. Think of quantitative research as a means of gathering accurate and reliable numerical data. Once all of the numerical data have been collected, we can then apply a wide variety of tests, assessments, analysis, and predictive applications to that data. This is where the value of quantitative research shines through—the interpretation of the numerical data collected. A host of analytical processes can be applied to numerical information—most to predict outcomes based on probabilities or to determine correlations among elements (**variables**) within the event being studied.

A simple example of a quantitative research endeavor would be to examine the likelihood of a coin coming up heads with each successive flip. If we were to begin the experiment by flipping a coin, we could measure the result by assigning a "1" to a heads result and a "0" to a tails result. By flipping the coin repeatedly, we can gather data in "1's" and "0's" for each of the events. After a prescribed number of events (say 100), we can then analyze our data. We may find that in 52 of the events (coin flips) we discovered that it came up heads (as indicated by 52 number "1's") and 48 times it came up tails. We can then apply the rules of probability statistics to these results to see if there was another explanation for the results other than chance. Probability laws dictate that the chance of a coin coming up heads or tails with each flip is 50 percent for each of the two outcomes. Our results of 52 percent and 48 percent are very close, and using statistical analysis we might find that our results are well within the range of probabilities.

A more thorough understanding of the principles and applications of probability statistics is outside the scope of this chapter. Interested readers should consider the references at the end of the chapter. It is also important to note that many software packages can execute very complex statistical analyses on data within a very short period of time. In fact, many users of these applications have a limited understanding of *how* they work—as long as the results are reliable, that's what matters to them. It may come as a surprise to many that you may already own a powerful statistical analysis software application: Microsoft Excel, which has a fairly diverse and useful collection of statistical applications embedded within it.

In summary, quantitative research is very valuable and has an important place in research in general. You may, or may not, find this approach to be useful in your analysis of a problem or opportunity. Knowing about it and how to apply it, though, are essential elements of research.

Qualitative Design

This research approach obviously has much less to do with numbers than with qualities (Remember: *qual*ity is a description of a characteristic, thus *qual*itative is descriptive in nature). To use the previous example, if we wanted to measure the size of the coin, the color of the coin, and the composition of the coin, we could apply numerical values to that research (quantitative design). But if we wanted to measure the beauty of the coin (how it makes us feel), that would necessitate descriptions of qualities of the coin—not an easy application to quantitative design. Instead, we'll consider a **qualitative design** approach so we can gather data about the qualities of the coin.

Qualitative research has been well established in the social sciences for a long time, but it is gaining increasing popularity in other disciplines as well (including the sciences). As researchers and analysts, we are finding more and more often that qualitative research can play a very important role in understanding a problem or opportunity. In fact, it is likely that you will find this approach to be more useful in discerning the underlying nature of most problems you will encounter in your EMS system or organization. Granted, some quantitative research may also be necessary to help elucidate the problem, but the larger component of inquiry is likely to be qualitative in nature.

The methods often employed in qualitative design include observation of subjects (either as a known observer or disguised as a participant), interviewing subjects (either individually or in a focused group), conducting surveys and questionnaires, case studies of an illustrative example, and a process known as **content analysis** where the written words are analyzed. Although other methodologies fall into the category of qualitative design, those mentioned here are the ones we'll focus on in this chapter.

Since qualitative research focuses on qualities of a subject or event, it could be argued that this approach is more subjective in nature — what one considers beautiful, appropriate, useful, pleasant, or even effective may be perceived differently by someone else. As such, qualitative research has long been regarded as less robust or meaningful. This mind-set has begun to change. Many people consider qualitative results to be just as meaningful and robust as their quantitative counterpart. Again, it's all about perception. The qualities that can be derived through qualitative methods cannot be obtained otherwise and, with proper attention to design and methods, can be every bit as revealing as the quantitative approach. As you complete this chapter, explore the different methods and see for yourself — both are quite valuable.

Mixed Methods Design

If one were to combine the two designs (quantitative and qualitative), you would create a mixed approach that carries the benefits of both approaches (and some of the limitations, of course): **mixed methods design**. As might be intuitive, this approach will likely be the best approach since it leverages the advantages of both designs. Many researchers share this perspective. To combine the quantitative design with the qualitative design enables the gathering of information that could not otherwise be obtained. You may choose to conduct both quantitative and qualitative research concurrently (at the same time), or you may elect to conduct them sequentially. Either way, this would likely render a more inclusive and

meaningful analysis and probably a more accurate result. Researchers are increasingly embracing this approach above all others — and you are encouraged to do the same. With any problem or opportunity, consider what elements of a quantitative approach and what elements of a qualitative approach could be applied and combined in your analysis.

PURPOSE

Research can also be categorized by purpose — that is, the intended reason for conducting the research. Generally, the three most recognized purposes for research are description, exploration, and explanation (Babbie, 2013). Usually, only one of these categories of research purpose is conducted at a time. If there is a need to conduct more than one, it is usually done sequentially, not concurrently. Here, we'll examine each of these.

Descriptive Research

In descriptive research, the investigator is attempting to provide observable or recordable details that help one to understand the nature of what is being researched. It is not necessarily an attempt to determine the cause of the problem or opportunity but, rather, the nature of it. It often answers the questions "What?" and "When?" and "Where?" Descriptive research is often the first type of research conducted when two or more types are conducted so as to gain a better understanding of the problem before delving deeper into causes or relationships among factors.

Examples of descriptive research are many. One example that many EMS providers may be familiar with is the annual EMS Salary and Workplace Survey conducted by *JEMS* (Greene and Wright, 2012). This endeavor typically presents to the readers a variety of details associated with EMS employment across the nation: compensation, benefits, types of shifts, and so on. Since it *describes* all of the details submitted by the participants of the survey, it is considered descriptive in nature.

Descriptive research is often regarded as essential to understanding a problem since it employs scientific methods and strict data collection methodologies to arrive upon the necessary information. As such, it is accurate and reliable and helps to inform the researcher or problem solver as to what additional research may be necessary. For this reason, it often represents the initial phase of research for analysis. Most descriptive research is qualitative in nature.

Exploratory Research

Exploratory research likely represents the majority of research endeavors. It is intended to inform the researcher of a new or unfamiliar event, a relationship between two or more factors underlying a problem, or the cause of a set of circumstances. Exploratory research tends to ask "Who?" and "How?" It will likely be one of the most important tools in your analysis of EMS system problems or opportunities. By its very nature, it is designed to discover hidden aspects or factors of a situation or event.

An example of a circumstance in which exploratory research would be best applied is trying to understand what types of EMS delivery systems exist in your state or region and how frequently each occurs. Another example is discovering how other EMS systems have adjusted to unanticipated drug shortages.

Exploratory research may be quantitative in nature (such as determining how many agencies follow this practice or what the frequency of an event is), but it is often qualitative in its use of interviews, surveys, and focus groups. This type of research is most suitable for inquiries regarding qualities (such as

"How is this done?" or "What is the current practice?" or "What is the structure of EMS delivery?"). Exploratory research may also comprise an initial investigation in anticipation of future research.

Explanatory Research

In this form of research, the intent is to explain events or relationships among two or more factors. It answers the question "Why?" This form of research may very well be the most probing and the most intense. It tries to get to the bottom of problems and opportunities so that one can better understand their nature and the reason for their existence. In summary, explanatory research often seeks to understand the causal factors behind these events and may be the most conclusive of research types analyzing EMS problems.

An example of explanatory research would be a study explaining why current reimbursement rates do not satisfy expenditure needs. A second example is the exploration of the motivating factors behind the perceived need to expand EMS services to neighboring communities. Explanatory research often represents the second phase of research, following either descriptive or exploratory research, but it may stand alone as an investigative endeavor.

Understanding why you need to conduct research for analysis (the purpose) and which of the three research types are best suited for this purpose will help you immensely in properly designing the research to render the best possible solutions. Much of the success in the entire analytical process is dependent on correct decisions along the way. Proper research design is one of the most critical.

METHOD

In this chapter, we will reduce the method of research to a simplified aspect and examine two broad, but distinctively different, approaches.

Methods of research can span a wide variety of procedural and design types, but we will focus only on two general categories: scientific method and social research method.

Scientific Method

In scientific research, the investigator typically conducts experiments in a highly controlled environment and assigns treatments or interventions to the subject in a very tightly managed manner to ensure no outside influences. This approach to research is perhaps the most reliable as it attempts to eliminate any extraneous influences to the outcome. Scientific inquiry often begins with a hypothesis that is offered to explain a phenomenon or event. Much of the clinical research conducted in medicine is of this type.

Researchers conducting this type of scientific inquiry are said to be using **experimental design**. This form of research attempts to control for any and all unwanted influences. One method that helps to ensure validity in results is to invoke a random assignment of subjects to the control and treatment groups. This will help eliminate any variances in results due to chance. A time-honored text authored by Campbell and Stanley, 1963, has established the design foundation for much of this type of study. Interested readers should consider this and other resources in the references at the end of this chapter.

An alternative approach to this scientific design is what is referred to as **quasi-experimental design**. This approach is almost identical to experimental design, but it lacks the random assignment feature. Often, this deficiency is not elective but necessary. It is always more favorable to randomly assign treatments to subjects, but sometimes that is not possible. For example, if one were researching the effects of a new drug on a rare disease, it would be difficult to anticipate when a patient will present with that disease, so random assignment may be impossible. It

then becomes acceptable to treat all patients with the particular disease with the new drug and account for the lack of randomness in treatment. Quasi-experimental design research is a very common approach and has great value in research.

Both the experimental and quasi-experimental approaches play a major role in the clinical application of research in EMS and emergency medicine. The developing trend is to ensure that every EMS professional has at least a general understanding of scientific inquiry and participates in meaningful research to grow the profession.

When applying scientific methods research to clinical data, be sure to comply with any and all established ethical standards. Unlike scientific research in a laboratory, when studying the treatment result or behavior of humans, an additional ethical concern exists. Patients in studies (referred to as subjects) are protected, by a host of ethical standards, from release of personal information, unethical treatments, unexplained risk, and undue complications. These ethical standards are typically implemented, enforced, and monitored by an **institutional review board (IRB)** or a human subject review committee. These oversight bodies often reside at institutions of higher learning (universities and colleges) and serve a critical role in protecting human rights and well-being. Be sure to discuss any patient-based study with the members of an IRB before proceeding with any element of a study.

Social Research Method

For the purposes of EMS system and organization problem analysis, the most applicable approach has its foundation in social research methods. Often, when inquiring as to why an event occurred or what the nature of a problem is, we cannot control the environment, nor can we randomly assign interventions to measure the outcome. By the same perspective, we also cannot expect to measure all outcomes numerically but must rely, at least somewhat, on qualitative measures. For these reasons, taking a social research approach is often most suitable in EMS analysis. As mentioned, qualitative research methods and social inquiry are becoming increasingly embraced by scientific investigators and will serve well as a means of problem resolution in EMS.

Side Bar

Clinical Research in EMS

Much research in EMS is clinical in nature. The articles that appear in peer-reviewed journals are most often about scientific research that focuses on treatment of illnesses or injuries or describes a diagnostic approach. These forms of research differ somewhat from investigational studies into EMS systems or organizational operations.

In clinical research, a quantitative approach is more common, often with randomized controlled trials (RCTs) or control groups, or blinded studies. These types of studies rely heavily on statistical probabilities to predict outcomes (often referred to as causal inferences). To better understand these types of research, a course in research methods is strongly recommended. In addition, a good reference text to better understanding these types of studies is *Studying A Study & Testing A Test: Reading Evidence-Based Health Research*, 6th edition, by Richard K. Riegelman (Philadelphia: Lippincott Williams & Wilkins, 2013).

Social research methods come in many forms and serve many purposes. Some of the more prevalent social research methods that may prove useful in analyzing an EMS problem or opportunity include the following:

- **Observation.** In this approach, the researcher observes the behavior and activities of the subjects in their natural setting. The observer may be a known researcher, collecting information through observation, or be disguised as a participant—known as a participant-observer. In either case, information is gathered strictly by observation.

- **Interviews.** This approach is very popular and productive. It involves questioning the subjects on specific topics to reveal the information necessary to understand the phenomenon or event. Often the questions are scripted and the conversations are recorded for later analysis. However, some forms of interviews are less formal and allow for contemporaneous discourse (qualitative interviews). Interviews are a great way to learn more about a situation or problem from another's point of view; however, it can be a lengthy process if you need to interview many people, one person at a time.

- **Focus group interviews.** Conducting **focus group interviews** is a way to expedite the data collection process from single-person interviews. In focus group interviews, individuals who have a common association (perhaps they work together, share the same problem that is being investigated, or all hold a similar job title) are gathered together and interviewed collectively. In this manner, many perspectives can be gathered at once. Clearly, one of the drawbacks of this approach is a condition known as group think. In group think, individuals begin to formulate their own opinions based on what others have already expressed, which tends to corrupt the data collection process by creating a homogenous response.

- **Surveys.** Another very popular and effective method of data collection are surveys (the actual survey questionnaire is often referred to as a survey instrument). Surveys can be oral (asking questions of the subjects), written (completing a paper or online survey form), or telephonic (asking questions of a subject over the telephone). In any case, the survey must be properly structured and administered under some degree of control. Survey instrument development is a subject worth learning, and courses dedicated to this purpose are available, including online courses. Most investigative inquiries involve some level of surveying individuals—it is a good idea to learn how best to develop proper survey instruments.

• **Case studies.** A case study in an exhaustive investigation into one or several exemplary cases of a particular problem or phenomenon. Somewhat unlike the traditional case studies used in EMS education where salient elements of a patient case are presented to inform participants, case studies in social research involve an exhaustive investigation into every possible detail that might hold some relevance to the problem. Case studies of this type are usually quite lengthy and involve multiple aspects of investigation, ultimately resulting in a comprehensive written report.

These approaches represent the more common forms of social research inquiry, and most will prove useful in your investigation of an EMS problem or opportunity. We will discuss some of these social research methods in more detail under the "Data Collection" section of this chapter.

It is not uncommon to combine several methods to fully explore and reveal the underlying problem. The more methods you employ in your analysis the more information you gain—but the greater the investment of time and resources and the more complex your analysis becomes. It is often beneficial to employ only one or two methods that appear to be the most revealing and leave the remainder for a later phase of inquiry if it becomes necessary.

TIME DIMENSION

How the research is conducted with regard to time is another important consideration in choosing what category of research you will employ. Generally, research designs may one of two time-related aspects: cross-sectional or longitudinal.

Cross-sectional Research

Research that is cross-sectional examines an event or phenomenon at one moment in time—it is somewhat like a snapshot of circumstances. For example, if you wanted to know how many members of your organization are paramedics, how many are EMTs, and how many are Advanced EMTs, you could survey the organization's current membership population. That would reveal, for that moment in time, how many in your organization hold each credential. Obviously, those numbers will change over time, but for that moment you have the needed information.

Cross-sectional research relies on the presumption that what is learned at that moment in time will be representative of what will be found at other moments in the time line, or at least it will be reasonably close. This approach is often satisfactory and can be quite revealing.

Longitudinal Research

By comparison, longitudinal research measures values over a period of time and is a continuous process. Most often, longitudinal research can be concurrent, retrospective, or prospective. **Concurrent research** begins measuring values of a variable beginning with the time the research starts and ends at a predetermined time. That is, the research is going on as the data are being collected concurrently. This is most commonly employed when combining quantitative methods with qualitative methods in the research design (mixed methods approach).

Retrospective research examines values of variables from the past. Known variables are searched for in documents, recordings, videos, or some form of permanent recordkeeping process. This approach relies on the presumption that such variables were previously recorded and can be obtained by reviewing the older records. A lot of empirical research is conducted retrospectively and is often the foundation for continued research in either concurrent or prospective approaches.

In **prospective research,** the recording of values of sought-after variables occurs at the beginning and ending of some predetermined future time. As the researcher, you are looking to the future for the information you seek. This is one way of confirming that the perceived problem actually does exist or that your implemented solution is actually effective (by conducting a prospective analysis).

Figure 3.2 graphically compares what the time elements of a cross-sectional and a longitudinal research study may look like. In the cross-sectional study, events were measured in the first month of 2007 and are represented at the time these events occurred. In the longitudinal study, the same events were measured beginning 1999 and recorded continuously until 2010. Fluctuations in the frequency (or nature) of the events that occurred in 2000 or

2005, for example, would be measured in the longitudinal study, whereas the cross-sectional study would not include them.

In addition to the *direction* of the time dimension (retrospective, concurrent, and prospective), other qualities of longitudinal research design may be considered. For example, perhaps you wanted to follow paramedic graduates to see how well they maintained their proficiencies in endotracheal intubation. By following all of the recent paramedic graduates (who may have come from different educational programs) for a specified period of time (perhaps one year), you are examining a cohort: individuals with a common statistical factor for research purposes (in this case, recent graduation). This is known as a **cohort study**. A similar model would be a **panel study**; instead of following any recent paramedic graduates, you would follow specific individuals from a particular paramedic graduating class for a predetermined period of time.

If, by comparison, you were to examine a specific characteristic or trait of a number of subjects over a given period of time, regardless of whether or not they have a similar

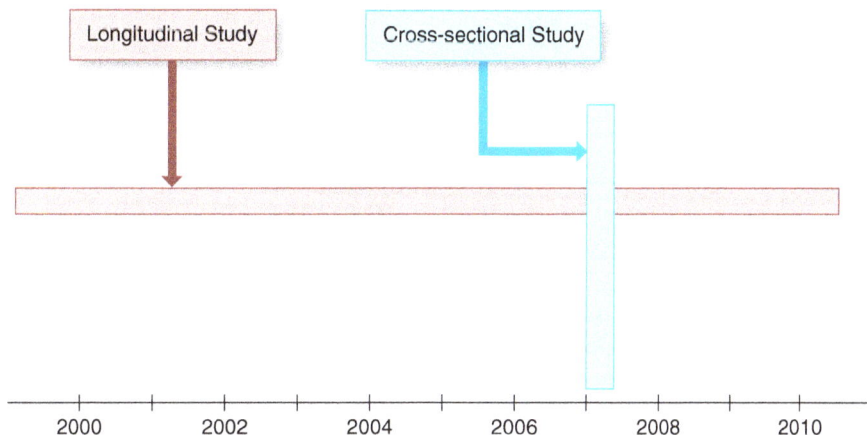

FIGURE 3.2 ■ Time-dimension perspective on research.

origin or common bond, you would likely be conducting a **trend study**. In a trend study, you follow the individuals who possess some characteristic that you are trying to study over a period of time and who have no commonality among themselves otherwise. An example would be looking at endotracheal intubation success rates of all paramedics, regardless of when they graduated.

In general, longitudinal studies are more revealing and, thus, more valuable forms of research. However, they are also more difficult to execute, more time-consuming, and certainly more expensive. One famous example of a longitudinal cohort study is the Framingham Heart Study. This study, begun in 1948, followed 5,209 individuals living in Framingham, Massachusetts, and sought to discover the contributing factors to cardiovascular heart disease. Much has been learned about cardiovascular disease from this study, but the expense associated with it is in the billions of dollars (Framingham Heart Study, 2013). Cross-sectional studies are easier to execute, less expensive, and useful in providing preliminary information that may lead to a longitudinal study in the future.

These represent some of the most common forms of categorization of research designs. Other forms are variations that may prove to be useful in your problem analysis.

OTHER IMPORTANT CONSIDERATIONS IN RESEARCH DESIGN

In addition to the category decisions, there are other important considerations when designing research for analysis. Each of the following aspects should be closely considered for any type of research to be employed; some have greater importance than others depending on the category of research being considered.

IDIOGRAPHIC VERSUS NOMOTHETIC EXPLANATION

Most individuals think of research as a means of determining every factor that causes a certain event or phenomenon to occur. This is a reasonably well-defined form of research known as **idiographic explanation**. Idiographic explanation exhaustively examines, based on one or several cases or examples, all of the factors that may cause a certain event or phenomenon. It is certainly an effective and useful form of research, but the investigator must choose representative cases to explain similar phenomena. By comparison, **nomothetic explanation** strives to find the most prevalent factors that cause most of the events or phenomena to occur. The simplest manner in which to view these two forms of research is this: Idiographic explanation is an exhaustive view of the many factors of representative cases that helps us to understand the event, and nomothetic explanation examines only several causative factors and uses probabilities to predict the likelihood that these are responsible for most similar events.

The nomothetic approach is more similar to the scientific method whereby statistical probabilities are used to determine **causality** (the factors that create the event or phenomenon). To understand causality, one must consider the concept of variables.

VARIABLES

Variables are representative factors that may influence the event or phenomenon that is under study. Each variable has associated with it attributes or values that characterize it. For example, if color was a variable, then green, blue, red, brown, and so on are the attributes or values of that variable color.

To put this into an EMS perspective, consider a study that endeavors to identify the underlying pathophysiology of patients with complaints of respiratory difficulty. Some of the variables that you may want to consider are skin color, lung sounds, pulse oximetry readings, $PETCO_2$ readings, patients' chief complaints, and vital signs (there are obviously many more). Each of these variables has a list of attributes or values associated with them:

- Skin color: pale, pink, reddened, blue, ashen, splotchy, and so on
- Lung sounds: clear, crackles, rhonchi, wheezes, friction rubs, and so on
- Pulse oximetry readings: above 98 percent, above 92 percent, below 92 percent (This variable can be continuous in that an actual number can be assigned to it that ranges anywhere from 0 to 100.)
- $PETCO_2$ readings: above 45 mm Hg, between 35 mm Hg and 45 mm Hg, and below 35 mm Hg (Again, this could be a **continuous variable** if so desired.)
- Patients' chief complaints: shortness of breath, labored breathing, dizziness, chest pain, nausea, and so on
- Vital signs: blood pressure measurements, pulse measurements, breathing measurements, temperature measurements, and so on

As you can see, selecting variables in a study is an extremely important task and can become quite extensive. For this reason, we try to be very selective about which variables are chosen in order to ensure relevance, importance, and ease of acquisition.

In our example, these variables will help to explain the underlying cause of the patient's breathing difficulties. Each of these variables will likely differ among patient subjects, and the combination values of these variables will help inform us as to the possible correlation with the cause of breathing problems. Because each of these contributes to the respiratory problem and can occur independently of each other, we regard each as an **independent variable**. That is, a patient can have shortness of breath and not have abnormal lung sounds, or

can have pink or blue skin color, or can also have a high $PETCO_2$ reading.

If you think about what we are trying to examine (the cause of respiratory difficulty), we discover that even the cause of respiratory difficulty is a variable and can have several possible attributes or values.

- Causes of respiratory difficulty: lung infection (pneumonia), pulmonary edema, asthma, emphysema, and so on

The difference between this variable (causes of respiratory difficulty) and the other independent variables is that the nature of the respiratory difficulty is *dependent* on the existence of the other (independent) variables (if we've chosen our independent variables correctly). That makes the causes of respiratory difficulty the **dependent variable**. To simplify things, we often refer to the independent variable as IV and the dependent variable as DV. Also, we can assign labels to each of the variables so that we don't have to write each one out every time. The following could be our variable list:

- Dependent variable (DV): Cause of respiratory difficulty—Resp
- Independent variables (IVs):
  - Skin color—SC
  - Lung sounds—LS
  - Pulse oximeter readings—SaO_2
  - $PETCO_2$—PET
  - Patients' chief complaints—CC
  - Vital signs—VS

Furthermore, to illustrate the relationships between the dependent and independent variables, we can construct the following simple formula:

$$Resp = SC + LS + SaO_2 + PET + CC + VS$$

This simple construct denotes that the dependent variable (causes of respiratory difficulties) is result of a combination of the independent variables. Theoretically, there are numerous other factors that haven't been considered in this simplistic model (including considerations for error), but the principles remain.

Criteria for Variable Selection

Yet another important aspect in selecting our variables is particularly important when considering the nomothetic approach. The variables chosen must have relevance and contribute toward the discovery of the dependent variable. Three criteria help to determine this: correlation, time order, and nonspuriousness.

Correlation means that the chosen variable must have some direct influence on the outcome. Typically, this relationship is direct and proportional (but it doesn't need to be) such that when the variable is present, it causes the outcome that we are seeking, and when the variable is present to a greater degree, the outcome is affected proportionally. Using our previous example, the presence of abnormal lung sounds is correlated with underlying respiratory disease. That is, when the lung sounds are more prevalent (greater), the acuity of the respiratory disease is likely more severe as well. It is probably obvious that abnormal lungs sounds can correlate to other events, but it still remains valid that there exists a correlation between the two variables that we are investigating.

Some variables are strongly correlated (have a greater direct influence or create a greater magnitude of change in the outcome variable), and some are weakly correlated. It is important to try to identify the strongly correlated variables. In nomothetic explanation design, the variables that are found to be correlated with the outcome variable and their strength of correlation can be estimated through statistical analysis of fairly large collections of data. This process represents one of the most valuable and powerful attributes of the statistical software used in research and analysis.

It is important to note that correlation, in and of itself, does not produce causality but is merely one criterion that is important to coexist with the others. It is possible for a variable to coexist with another (and even for them to change in concert with each other) but have no direct influence on one another.

Time order is another somewhat obvious criterion for proper variable selection. In **time order**, we are referring to the condition that the variable under consideration *must* precede the occurrence of the outcome variable (DV) in time. Put another way, the cause must precede the effect. This relationship can go either way; the DV can create the IVs and vice versa. What is important is that one must precede the other to create causality. In our example, the vital signs, the presence of adventitious lung sounds, abnormal pulse oximetry and $PETCO_2$ readings, and chief complaints are all a product of the presence of the underlying respiratory disease. Some causality remains since the underlying respiratory disease must precede the presence of the independent variables.

Time order can become a fairly complex relationship, particularly if there is more than one dependent variable. It is not as important to determine direction of the time order (which one occurs first) but, rather, that it actually does exist between the two (or more) variables.

The last criterion, nonspuriousness, may be the most difficult to understand and often offers some challenges to the analyst. **Nonspuriousness** means that the effect the variable of interest has on the outcome variable is directly linked and not a product of some other, outside factors. This criterion is somewhat related to correlation except that correlation does not specify that the relationship must be direct and unique. Nonspuriousness requires that another, third variable (that is often unknown) isn't also responsible for the influence on the outcome variable. As one might imagine, this is somewhat difficult to ensure. For that reason, we try our best to ensure nonspuriousness in our variable selection, but we also accept that some degree of spuriousness might creep in. In our example, one might ask "Does the variable vital sign or pulse oximeter readings affect skin color?" Clearly, that answer is "Yes." If the blood pressure is low and/or the pulse oximeter readings are low, the skin color will change accordingly. This relationship demonstrates a level of spuriousness among those variables. However, they are still meaningful because they have a strong correlation to the outcome variable and also exhibit time order.

To develop an awareness of these three criteria, it might be a good exercise to think of other relationships among variables that would challenge you to identify the strengths of these criteria in those relationships. For example, do years of experience correlate well with success in endotracheal intubation? Or does the distance from the station to the origin of the call relate to patient outcome (morbidity or mortality)? Some of these relationships might be the actual basis of our investigation.

OPERATIONALIZATION

As important as the concept of operationalization is, it is often a source of confusion and misunderstanding among new researchers. For that reason, we'll attempt to simplify this concept and offer a few examples.

Simply put, **operationalization** is the process that yields the data necessary for each variable. Thus, the relationship between variables and operationalization is critical. Once your variables are selected, you must decide how to operationalize or measure them. Let's say your variable is "The public sentiment

about your EMS agency expanding services into the neighboring community." This would be an important variable in our analysis of whether or not to expand services. But how would you measure that variable? Perhaps you would distribute a survey or questionnaire that asks (among other questions) the subject's opinion about the expansion. Or maybe you would interview some representative individuals or even conduct focus group interviews. Each of these approaches represents the operationalization of the variable "public sentiment."

Each time you select a variable, you should contemplate how it will be operationalized. If you struggle with a methodology to operationalize a variable, then your effort at analysis may be futile. Operationalization must be valid (truly produces the data you seek), reliable (is consistent in producing the same information when applied), and relatively simple to execute (does not create investigational blocks in the process). This is yet another example of the importance of forethought in research design or analytical development. Figure 3.3 presents some examples of the concept of operationalization.

As one might surmise from the examples in Figure 3.3, operationalization can become a complex and possibly unmanageable endeavor. In fact, some of the operationalization processes noted have the potential to stand alone as an initial data collection process for the next phase of analytical investigation.

UNITS OF ANALYSIS

The concept of **units of analysis** represents another component in research and analysis design that challenges understanding at times. Again, let's try to keep this concept simple. Units of analysis are those entities that we use to measure the operationalization of our variables. They are the elements that we must examine or

Variable	Examples of Operationalization
Vital signs	Collecting measurements from previous patient care reports (if retrospective study)
Revenue generated by a 0.1% tax hike	Examination of public tax documents at local tax office; or interview city clerk's office personnel
Cost of acquiring a new LifePak 15	Perusing the Internet for the manufacturer's website, or talking with the company's representative
Benefit of acquiring a new LifePak 15	Examining peer-reviewed journal articles for impact of 12-lead electrocardiography on patient outcomes, or conducting a literature search on the lives saved through prehospital EKG and defibrillation interventions
Public acceptance of instituting community paramedic services	Interview hospital leadership, doctor's offices, and clinics; focus group surveys of aged groups; survey home health care nurses; anonymous surveys of paramedical staff

FIGURE 3.3 ■ Examples of operationalization.

discern to render the process of measurement so that we can assign a value to our variable. They are, in fact, what we will study. The nature of the challenge in understanding this concept is that we tend to become too specific or narrow in our consideration of units of analysis.

For example, if we wanted to learn the sentiment of the general public regarding our proposed service expansion, we would want to interview local police, fire, and city administrative personnel. We would also want the perspective of the hospital staff, doctors, and similar health care providers. We may also want to interview members of the public in each of the communities. It's easy to begin to construct a lengthy list of professional types from whom we want an opinion, but what we are really seeking is the opinion of *individuals*. So, regardless of the role the person plays, the units of analysis are individuals. We can later label the variables as to their occupation if that becomes necessary.

Similarly, if we were to try to gather patient medical information from previous patient care reports to retrospectively obtain data for our analysis, then we would be examining *documents* as our unit of analysis. We often can identify the unit of analysis by reducing the element to the lowest common denominator. But we need to be careful to ensure that our unit of analysis accurately describes what we are studying. If we wanted the opinion of only paramedics in our research inquiry, then we would be examining a group of individuals and, thus, the unit of analysis would be *groups*, not individuals. Think of the units of analysis as units of observation or units of study—what it is that we will be looking at.

THEORETICAL STRUCTURE OF INQUIRY

How we plan to approach our inquiry and structure our analysis should be thought through from the very beginning. It is best to have an overall plan or approach to our investigation from the start. We will need to gain an overall perspective of our analysis and how we plan to accomplish our end goal. When doing so, we generally will be taking one of two approaches: either an inductive approach or a deductive approach.

Inductive Approach

An **inductive approach** involves gathering pieces of information (data) from observation, inquiry, surveying, or similar processes; compiling that information into an aggregate form; and interpreting it to formulate a general, all-inclusive explanation. It is best thought of as going from the particulars to the general. This approach is akin to inductive reasoning, thus the name. An example would be collecting all of the clinical findings of patients with respiratory difficulties, compiling all of that information, and inferring that it represents a particular respiratory pathology. A patient with difficulty breathing, wheezing, nonproductive cough, prolonged expiration, tachycardia, hypercapnia, and "shark-fin" capnograph (the *particulars*) leads one to suspect a patient with bronchial asthma (the *general*). Figure 3.4 depicts a conceptual model of an inductive approach to investigation.

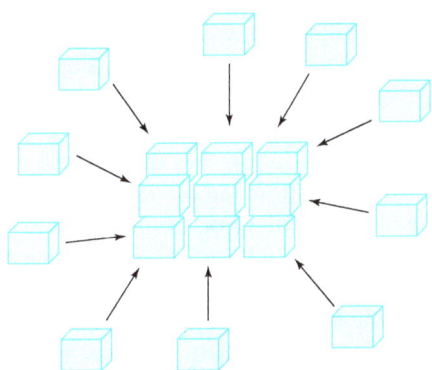

Deductive Approach

A **deductive approach** is the general method of considering an overall belief, theory, or explanation as to the cause of the event and searching out the details to verify its existence. It is best thought of as going from the general to the particulars (akin to deductive reasoning). To use the previous example, if you were to suspect that a person is having a bronchial asthma attack (the *general*), you would look for the details of evidence (the *particulars*). The child's mother may tell you that he has asthma, so you would look for the clinical findings of difficulty in breathing, wheezing, nonproductive cough, prolonged expiration, tachycardia, and hypercapnia with a "shark-fin" waveform on the capnograph. The conceptual representation of a deductive approach is also illustrated in Figure 3.4.

SOME FINAL THOUGHTS BEFORE BEGINNING THE DESIGN

Before beginning our research design for analysis, be sure to consider each of the following:

* What is the time line for completion? How much time is available to design the research, collect the data, conduct the analysis, and draw the necessary conclusions?

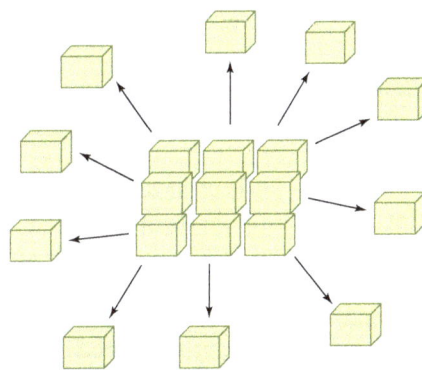

Inductive–from particulars to the general   **Deductive**–from the general to the particulars

FIGURE 3.4 ■ Inductive and deductive approaches.

- What are our resources? How much money is necessary to execute our plan? Do we have the supplies, the personnel, the necessary paperwork, and all of the required authorizations?
- What is the political climate for our analysis? Who are the stakeholders? Who are our clients? Who will benefit from the results? Will it harm any interested groups or entities?
- What other analyses might be necessary? Should there by a financial analysis? Should we conduct a cost-benefit analysis? What about an impact analysis?

These and other thoughts should be considered before we begin. We may not be able to address all considerations at the start (and some may need to be revised once we've begun our analysis), but we should be thinking of them throughout the analytical process. Jotting them down early in the process may help us to avoid some untimely errors or embarrassments later. By all means, keep an open mind and be flexible in your approach—especially in the beginning. You may start off convinced you have a solid plan, only to discover that your approach was wrong and you need to revise it midway through the process. That is the nature of research and analysis. As long as we abide by the rules and rigidly comply with research practices, we can still produce some very meaningful results.

CONDUCTING THE RESEARCH FOR ANALYSIS

Now that we have a fairly clear understanding of why the research methods are important and what the different types of research are, we are now ready to begin the process. Generally, this process is a step-by-step progression that concurs with the order described in the following subsections. It is possible, and acceptable, to alter the order when circumstances dictate that a variance in progression

is necessary, but those circumstances should be infrequent. It is best to try to follow the progression as follows.

PROBLEM IDENTIFICATION AND THE KEY RESEARCH QUESTION

Proper problem identification is the critical first step and has been discussed thoroughly in this chapter. Through our preliminary analysis of mind mapping, logic model development, literature searches, and contemplative thought, we already have verified the existence and nature of the problem, and so we begin our research for analysis.

To begin that process, we must translate our "problem" into a workable **key research question**. This simply is a process of formulating a question that, when answered, will specify the information needed to resolve the identified problem. For example, if our organization is faced with the prospect of coverage expansion into the neighboring community, the key research question may be "Is it feasible to expand services into the neighboring community?" Or if we've identified a problem with paramedics failing to properly recognize the underlying pathologies of respiratory distress, we could ask "How well do the paramedics recognize the differential pathologies of respiratory disease?" or "Why are the paramedics failing to recognize underlying pathologies of respiratory distress accurately?" As you might surmise, there can be more than one research question in a system analysis. What is important is that there is only one key research question and all other research questions are subsidiary or secondary to that principal key research question. Each **secondary research question** should modify or supplement the key research question.

The key research question is important as it guides the subsequent research process. Therefore, it must be representative of the problem, concise, focused, and answerable. If we were to pose the following key research question, "What is the ideal EMS delivery model for the United States?", we would be faced with a nearly insurmountable research task. It is too broad and would require an incredible amount of resources to investigate. (Note: There are alternatives to how this question could be investigated that would make it much more manageable. For example, one could conduct a qualitative inquiry on "What is the predominant consensus among EMS professionals and administrators in [select a geographic region] as to the ideal EMS delivery model?" At least that key research question could be reasonably answered.)

The importance of the key research question cannot be overemphasized. In fact, it is not uncommon for a researcher to have crafted the key research question, already designed the research, collected data, and begun analysis only to discover that the key research question is not adequate. The researcher would then go back and revise the key research question and either modify the design, data collection, and analysis or start all over—it is *that* important.

SELECTING AND IMPLEMENTING YOUR RESEARCH DESIGN

At this stage, we have been presented with what is perceived to be a problem or opportunity for analysis. This should always begin with considerations as to what types of research are necessary and appropriate.

We should be asking ourselves whether the research should be qualitative in nature or quantitative in nature, or both. Think about what it is you're trying to accomplish. Are you trying to understand the nature of the problem, as in an exploratory investigation? Or are you trying to explain why the problem exists, as in an explanatory purpose? Or is it strictly descriptive in nature? Furthermore, would a scientific or a social inquiry approach be more

appropriate? By the way, for the purposes of analysis, most problems are conducive to a social research approach.

We should also consider the time dimension in our initial design thoughts. Can this be done retrospectively, or do we need to be prospective in our approach? Or can we simply gather a snapshot of the situation through a cross-sectional design?

Give a lot of thought to how you would ultimately envision this design for analysis. Having a mental picture of what it will look like in the end helps immensely in the initial design stages. However, avoid becoming married exclusively to that design. In research, it is quite common to revise and redesign a developing research model. Keep an open mind and remain flexible in your initial design.

CHOOSING YOUR VARIABLES, METHODS OF OPERATIONALIZATION, AND UNITS OF ANALYSIS

Now that we have an overall plan for the research design, we should now proceed to identify our variables. The first variable will likely be the dependent variable: what it is you're trying to uncover. It might be feasibility of expansion of services, acquisition of new equipment, impact of revenue reductions, or a substantive change in call volume. Whatever the problem is that you're trying to understand or resolve, the dependent variable should inform that aspect.

With the dependent variable selected, begin to identify all of the possible independent variables that *might* influence the dependent variable. Your initial list should be long and inclusive—you can pare it down later. Think about all of the possible factors or qualities that might influence the dependent variable. At this stage, don't worry too much about correlation, time order, or nonspuriousness—you can revise them shortly. It is more important to generate an all-inclusive list initially and then proceed to eliminate those that are irrelevant, redundant, lacking the necessary criteria for variable selection, or immeasurable (some simply can't be measured).

Once you've identified all of your variables and have eliminated those that you can, you should label those that are of interest with brief, but descriptive, names. The shorter the label, the more manageable they are.

Now take each individual variable and think about how you will measure it. What process will be necessary for you to gain the information you'll need to satisfy that variable? This process of operationalization is important and deserves some time and consideration. Think about the easiest ways to measure the values of the variables and the methods that would be most accurate and reliable. Do this for each of the independent variables. If you cannot operationalize a variable, then you effectively cannot use it.

A word of caution is important here: If you have created a long list of variables and a fairly complex series of operationalization methods for them, you are likely facing an unmanageable endeavor in research analysis. Some of the best advice is to keep it simple—at least initially. If time allows, you can always go back and make your analysis more comprehensive by adding variables and/or operationalization processes.

Once you've identified your variables of interest and how you will operationalize them, consider what your units of analysis will be. What subjects, documents, sources, or records do you need to examine to derive the necessary data for each variable in order to conduct your analysis? Identifying your units of analysis early can also help you in your research design.

With your research design in mind, the variables selected, the methods of operationalization and the units of analysis identified, you are ready to start data collection. This is an exciting and often engaging aspect of your research for analysis.

DATA COLLECTION

How you plan to gather data is actually part of the research design and operationalization of the variables. If your design is qualitative and longitudinal in nature, you may have decided to collect data on your variable through surveys or perhaps interviews. This particular design aspect determines your data collection methods. When you get to this stage of the study, you'll probably already have a good idea as to what your data collection methods will be. The important goal to keep in mind is to conduct data collection within strict guidelines and procedural control to prevent corruption of data and maintain ensurances of validity.

Data collection comes in many forms. There are entire books and college courses dedicated to data collection methods. Here we will focus on some of the more common methods.

Surveys

If you plan to collect data via surveys and questionnaires, you are likely conducting a qualitative investigation. However, many quantitative inquiries can be accomplished via surveys as well. If you are conducting a paper survey, the document is considered a **data collection instrument**. It can be a series of questions that are open ended or several that ask for a quantitative response. If the survey instrument is asking the respondent to rate his response numerically on a scale, it is quantitative and probably uses a **Likert scale** for valuation. This often ranges from 1 to 5 in value, and the respondent chooses the number that most closely represents his choice. The benefit to this approach is that you can use statistical analysis to help interpret your results since subject responses are numerical. Figure 3.5 provides a simple example of the use of a Likert scale in a survey.

Otherwise, survey instruments may request a response of a word, several words, a

Please respond to each of the following questions by circling the value that most closely represents your level of agreement, from no agreement "1" to complete agreement "5."

Question	Disagree				Agree
1 Do you think your local emergency medical services agency should expand to provide coverage to the nearby communities?	1	2	3	4	5
2 I am willing to pay more in taxes to support the expansion of my local emergency medical services agency.	1	2	3	4	5

FIGURE 3.5 ■ Likert scale examples.

sentence, or even a short paragraph. Such survey instruments are typically used in qualitative investigations. Alternatively, the respondent may be asked to select from a list of choices, much like a multiple-question examination. If using survey instruments as a means of data collection appeals to you, you may want to purchase a book on how best to design them effectively.

Another form of surveying is via telephone—this is referred to as a **telephonic survey**. It is similar in approach to the traditional document survey, except that the investigator (or his designee) asks the questions

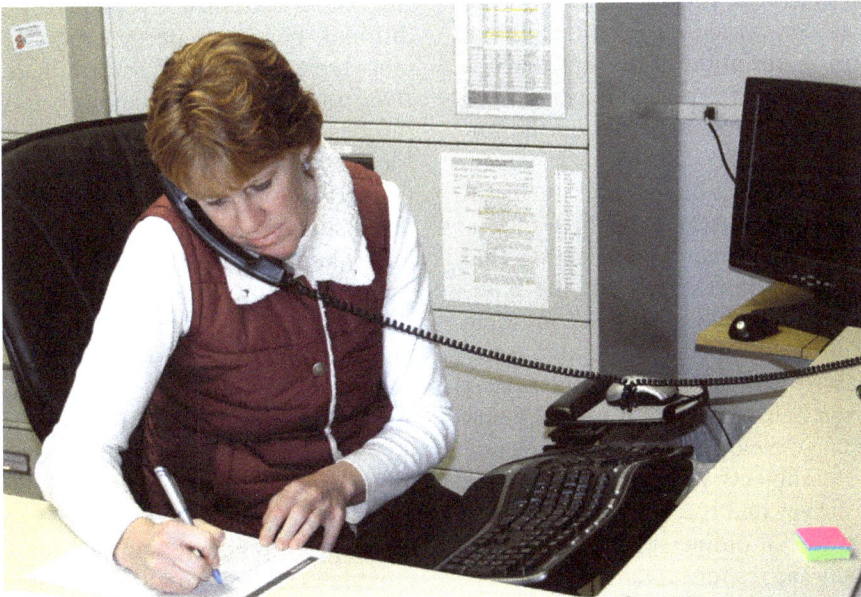

FIGURE 3.6 ■ Telephonic survey.

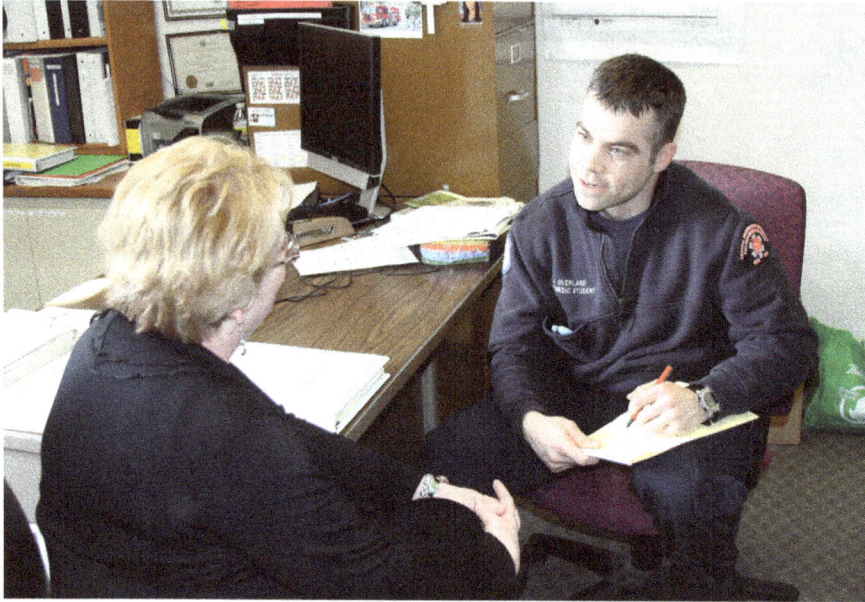

FIGURE 3.7 ■ Individual interview.

from the survey instrument and records the respondent's answers. Thereafter, the data are compiled as they would be for a traditional survey form. A variation of this approach is when the subject is interviewed in person and the interviewer records responses on the survey instrument.

Internet surveying has gained considerable popularity as a data collection instrument. There are commercial businesses that provide survey support services on the Internet at very reasonable rates and, in some cases, free of charge. For a reasonable price, they will assist you in building your survey and can even help distribute it to recipients. You often can develop the online survey and provide your subjects with the URL link to access the survey and record their responses. These commercial online survey companies will then tally the responses, categorize them, and provide some simple analysis of data.

Interviews

Interviews also come in several forms. The traditional, person-to-person interview is the most typical and familiar form. It is an effective tool and can engender uninhibited responses, but the method is time consuming for the researcher. An additional advantage of this format is that the interviewer can facilitate discussions and even pursue threads of dialogue that are germane to the investigation.

A variation of this means of data collection is group interviews, whereby more than one subject is interviewed. The group often exhibits some commonality (workplace, interest, similar role), and the discussion focuses on a singular topic. Group interviews are common in marketing strategies and are referred to as focus group interviews. Group interviewing is more efficient than person-to-person interviews but inaccurate information may be obtained due to participant dominance, group

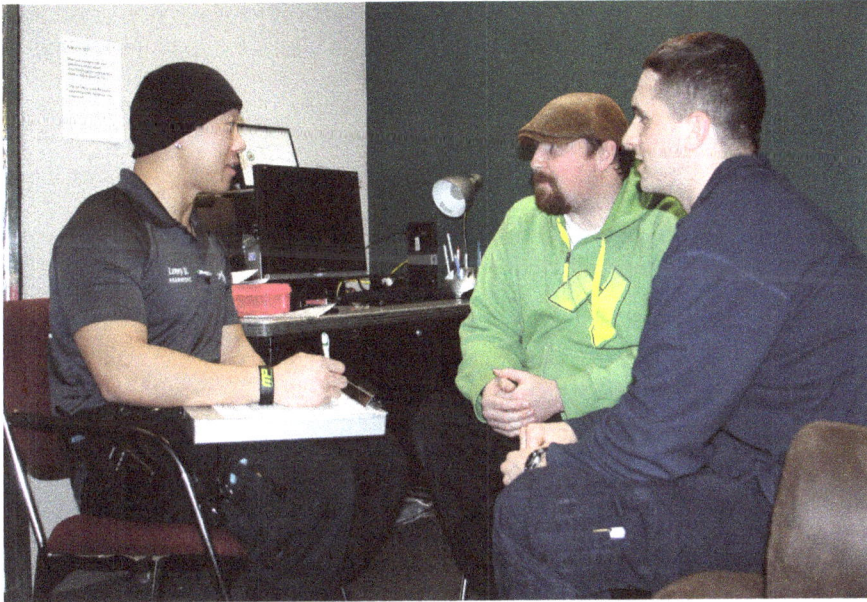

FIGURE 3.8 ▦ Focus group interview.

think, or individuals' inhibition in multiperson settings.

Interviews are an excellent method of gaining insight into a problem or gathering meaningful data. What one should not rely on is one's own memory for data collection. Interviews should be recorded (permission to record the subject should first be obtained) and the dialogue later transcribed for analysis. Only in this manner can accurate information be recorded. Digital recording devices are inexpensive and easily reusable. Video recording is another alternative, but it can be costly and difficult to manage by oneself. Despite digital or video recordings, always make a habit of taking notes during the interview—a practice that will prove useful for later reference.

Additional forms of interview methods can include telephonic, over the Internet, and via messaging. In any case, be sure to gather all necessary supplies before beginning the interview and always seek permission to interview the subject. It is generally best to maintain anonymity of the subject when collecting data via interviews.

Document Review

In some instances, you may need to review records or other documents to glean salient information from them. This process of data collection is very common in retrospective studies and can be very effective at a reasonably low cost. In collecting data in this manner, the investigator will assess the documents with a predetermined set of queries. To facilitate the process, these predetermined data elements, or fields, are compiled on a query form that is completed for each document reviewed. Sometimes the data recording sheet is a tick sheet on which information is confirmed, or the document can have a scale that enables the investigator to quantify the findings.

A similar approach would apply if a case study were to be conducted. Documentation of many aspects of the case would be necessary, and a reliable means of recording case findings is essential. Much of this takes the form of simple note taking and contextual analysis. More information regarding contextual analysis can be found in the "Data Analysis" section of this chapter.

Recording Quantitative Findings

Should your analysis involve some level of quantitative research, the numerical findings of your data collection should be systematically and precisely recorded in a clear and reliable manner. The documentation should stand up to scrutiny by others and be easily corroborated to ensure veracity of purpose and intent. Often, researchers will develop a data form beforehand to aid in the recording of information.

This information can then be entered into a data set electronically, either by transference or direct data entry. The data set should be compatible with whatever software application you will use for statistical analysis. For simple quantitative data analysis, this can be accomplished in a single step by entering the findings directly into a spreadsheet such as Microsoft Excel. Other software packages may require a different format.

ANALYSIS OF DATA

Now that the data have been collected, it is time to begin your analysis of the findings. For many researchers, this is the most exciting part, as what the analysis reveals is often not readily apparent simply by data collection. Analysis is a critical part of the research process as it determines the eventual outcome. For this reason, it must be conducted

with absolute precision and an unbiased methodology. Recognizing common errors in analysis or common threats to validity is very important to all researchers. Therefore, a brief discussion of some of the common errors and threats to validity follows.

Validity

Validity has its greatest relevance in quantitative analysis but also has many applications in sociological inquiry. Since there is considerable crossover, we will regard its application to both quantitative and qualitative research simultaneously, even though it may have greater application in one aspect than the other.

In general terms, validity is analogous to veracity. If we are attempting to discover information, gain a better understanding of a perceived problem, or consider alternative explanations to an event, we want to know the truth. To achieve that level of understanding relies heavily on deriving valid information, thus the correlation. In quantitative analysis, validity represents gaining the truth through the inference of the data collected. Similarly, in qualitative analysis, validity approximates the truth through multidimensional perspectives. Both types of analysis have similar foundations. Numerous resources discuss the philosophical aspects of validity in research. Readers are encouraged to consider some of the references listed at the end of this chapter.

Validity most likely has its greatest influence in the design of the research. If you have designed your research analysis well, validity becomes less of a concern. For that reason, knowing the types of validity and the common threats to validity is essential to designing your research.

Types of Validity and Threats to Validity

Research typically concerns itself with four forms of validity: internal validity, external validity, statistical conclusion validity, and construct validity. In this chapter, we will address internal and external validities and refer the reader to other sources for statistical conclusion validity and construct validity.

Internal validity can be thought of as "Did the process of investigation reveal the true nature of the problem or event?" To be reflective of the reality, our efforts at investigation must be devoid of any prejudice, bias, design error, or procedural mistakes. The data collected should demonstrate the actual nature of the problem or event under investigation. From a quantitative investigational perspective, internal validity centers on whether the observed results reflect the causal relationships between measured dependent and independent variables.

We began addressing internal validity when we considered the criteria for variable selection (correlation, time order, and nonspuriousness). However, there are more considerations than simply variable selection when ensuring internal validity. Some of the most important include these:

- **Selection bias**—not allowing subject or variable inputs to be chosen or included in the study by any external or prejudicial influences; making sure that selections are truly representative of the population under study; most often ensured by randomization of selection.
- **Experimenter (or inter-rater) bias**—when the individual conducting the data collection or observational assessment inadvertently behaves differently among subjects of the study. (When more than one person collects the data and each behaves differently among the subjects, it is termed inter-rater bias.)
- **Self-reporting bias**—when information is offered by the subject that is consciously or subconsciously altered to satisfy the expected responses to the inquiry
- **History effects**—when events that are occurring during the study could influence the outcome and even create the final results.

- **Attrition effects**—when subjects in the study drop out or withdraw, thereby creating erroneous outcomes that are not truly representative of the study population.
- **Maturation effects**—when subjects change over the duration of the study, resulting in changes in outcomes; most often associated with longitudinal studies.
- **Confounding effects**—when the dependent variable is altered or affected by an independent variable that is not identified or not regarded as relevant (often has some association with one of the independent variables); also known as a spurious condition.
- **Testing effects**—when the study results are altered simply by virtue of the test assessment itself; the process of testing actually alters the subject's behavior; related to the **Hawthorne effect** (when subject behavior is altered simply by the subject's knowledge that they are being studied).

Although there are more threats to internal validity than those listed here, these represent some of the most common or most damaging to the study process. When designing the research model, keep these threats in mind and design the data collection and variable selections to help avoid these problematic aspects.

Another form of validity is **external validity** or generalization. Simply put, external validity is the ability to apply the findings of the study from the select study population group to other, similar groups outside of the study. In other words, if you were to study an EMS system in Pennsylvania, would those results apply to EMS systems in Washington State? Or do the results from an isolated study have application to similar organizations or entities elsewhere geographically? This concept may even be applied to differences in organizational type and not just geography. Do the lessons learned from a study of private EMS delivery systems have applicability to public EMS delivery models?

External validity threats are common because it is often impossible to study a subject population broad enough to be representative of the entire target population. The costs associated with increasing the number of subjects and varying their geographic location as well as their agency types would be prohibitive. This is a recognized limitation in most studies.

Statistical Analysis

When conducting quantitative analyses, the numerical results are often responsive to statistical analysis. Statistical analysis is largely a matter of predicting outcomes based on probabilities and seeking statistical correlation among variables—particularly independent and dependent variables. For example, if in our earlier example of variable selections for underlying causes of respiratory distress, we were interested in to what extent abnormal breath sounds can be correlated with respiratory distress, we could conduct a statistical analysis of those two variables. Perhaps we found that in 78 percent of the cases of respiratory distress, abnormal lungs sounds were identified in the patient. To what extent are those two variables correlated, and does their occurrence result from chance? A statistical process is required to make those determinations.

Statistical analysis is beyond the scope of this chapter, and there are many reliable and effective textbooks and courses on that subject. If you anticipate becoming an earnest quantitative analyst, then you may want to investigate some of the more powerful statistical software packages such as SAS, Stata, or IBM-SPSS Statistics.

Content Analysis

When conducting qualitative research, some of the data most likely to be collected will be in written form. Interviews (individual or group), nonquantitative surveys, some document reviews, video or audio recording reviews, and journal article reviews can benefit from content analysis. Content analysis is the process of studying recorded communication (most often in written form). When you read an article, passage, or even a paragraph, you synthesize a general meaning of the context by assimilating the various messages it contains. This process of generalization and consolidation of information is important to rapid understanding while reading, but it may overlook even the most glaring points or repetitive concepts. In content analysis, the process demands a detailed and meticulous examination of the context to identify these points of interest and repeating themes.

Basically, the process begins by transcribing any audio or video recordings into written form. The analyst then begins the detailed process of reviewing each statement for an important point or topic of discussion. Those findings are abbreviated into one or two words and recorded (often in the margin of the text), and the process continues for the entire document. This process of identifying themes and repeating concepts is termed **coding** and requires a structured framework and clear definition of the concepts being sought. Coding in content analysis is a form of operationalization of variables. Figure 3.9 provides a simple example of a transcribed interview with content analysis and coding.

Content analysis can take two forms: **manifest content** and **latent content**. In manifest analysis, the analyst looks for a specific word or collection of words and records the frequency of occurrence in the document (and sometimes the context in which it appears). For example, if you were interested in determining what new diagnostic procedure your agency should invest in next, you may want to interview a number of emergency medicine physicians, experienced EMS practitioners, EMS educators, and some medical vendors. In the course of the interviews, you would audio-

Interviewer: "If you were given an unlimited budget, what types of equipment would you purchase for your ambulance?"

Respondent: "Well, that's difficult to say. I guess I would buy monitor defibrilla-tors since they are so expensive, or maybe some new technology."

Monitor defibrillators

Interviewer: "What kind of new technology would you consider?"

Respondent: "I don't know. I guess a Doppler. No, wait! I know. I would buy a portable ultrasound machine."

Doppler Portable ultrasound

Interviewer: "Do you mean a portable handheld ultrasound machine? How much do those cost?"

Respondent: "I'm not sure. Maybe ten thousand dollars. I'm really not sure."

$10,000

Interviewer: "Do you think it would be useful, perhaps save more lives?"

Respondent: "Yeah, probably. I've heard that you can identify abdominal hem-orrhage with those when you can't otherwise. It seems it would be very useful to find life-threatening problems in our patients as early as possible. It seems to me to be a good idea."

Abdominal hemorrhage

Interviewer: "Is that something that you see as paramedics using in the future?

Respondent: "I do. In fact, I heard that some agencies are using them right now. I'm sure it will be standard equipment in the near future—you know, when the technology gets better and the prices come down."

Price reductions

FIGURE 3.9 ■ Content analysis with coding.

record the interview and take notes. A prod-uct of those recorded interviews would be a transcription of the dialogue. You could then reread the interviews and "code" the occur-rences of any type of new diagnostic tool or intervention. By quantifying their occurrences you "manifest" their presence by a numerical frequency and may discover that prehospital ultrasonography is the most often mentioned innovative practice.

Latent content, by comparison, is a bit more investigative. Here you are looking for the underlying meaning of the discussion or written words, not the actual occurrences of words. This is clearly somewhat subjective and requires some level of interpretation, but it has great significance as most communication is more than simply a list of words strung together. There is hidden meaning in much of communi-cation and this "latent" content is often more important than the words themselves.

The process in latent content analysis is fundamentally the same—the analyst examines the document and records the interpreted ideas or principles in the margin, then exam-ines the results for relevance and occurrences. Once again, having a well-defined framework and clear definitions of concepts is important in any form of content analysis to ensure the validity of findings.

A number of software applications exist that facilitate content analysis and provide the necessary framework to ensure validity. How-ever, most simple content analysis can be completed manually, as described previously in this chapter.

Content analysis has several advantages and disadvantages. The advantages include the low cost associated with its use, the simplicity of the application, the ability to correct analysis midstream, and the fact that content analysis is done outside of the data collection process (outside the presence of the subject) and, as such, is unobtrusive. The disadvantages are that it is subject to threats of validity (particularly experimenter bias) and that it is limited to written documents or transcriptions.

INTERPRETATION OF ANALYSIS AND DRAWING CONCLUSIONS

Once all of the data are collected and the analysis is complete, the analyst must begin to make sense of it all. Some would argue that this is the easiest part since "the data speak for themselves." And, to a point, this is true. If designed well and structured correctly, the research should lead the analyst to the obvious conclusions. This is highly dependent on not only a proper design but also a careful selection of variables, methods of operationalization, units of analysis, and application of proper analytical methodologies. Your focus should be "Do the analytical results answer the key research question?" If so, then your interpretation and conclusions are fairly straightforward. If not, then either you must go back and redesign the study, reselect the correct variables and other parameters, and repeat the study; or render an incomplete interpretation and conclusion citing the deficiencies and limitations upfront.

Even research that is somewhat unsuccessful isn't meaningless; it still contributes to knowledge and understanding. If you've invested a considerable amount of time and effort into your analysis only to discover you haven't answered the key research question completely, you can still render a speculated interpretation and draw reasonable conclusions as long as you identify the deficiencies and limitations of the analysis. This will inform others and allow the process to be repeated with improved validity and reliability in the future.

■ PUTTING IT ALL TOGETHER AND THE NEXT STEP———————

At this point, we should begin to consider how to put all of this together. You may come to realize that much of the initial process is a bit amorphous and uncertain, but as you begin putting it together, it will take shape and have purpose. Be sure to follow the progressive steps as outlined in this chapter since each step informs and defines the subsequent steps. A summary of the steps is illustrated in Figure 3.10.

Remember, you may need to revise your research design as you progress through the process. In fact, you may even discover that your key research question may need revision. You may also find that needed variables are missing and must be included, or perhaps the operationalization process you've chosen is ineffective and another must be considered. The research process for analysis is a dynamic process and often undergoes some revision or refinement throughout.

For the purposes of analysis, this research component is clearly essential, but it may be inadequate. Although it structurally forms the foundation of the analytical approach, it may be insufficient in its analytical scope. For that reason, you will often need to consider additional elements of analysis—such as financial analysis, cost-benefit analysis, feasibility analysis, and impact analysis—to develop an effective solution to the problem or a clear course of action for a new opportunity. Many of these additional elements may have an equal or greater contribution toward resolution than the research approach itself. However, no conclusive decision should be made without considering all essential elements and integrating those elements in the final analysis.

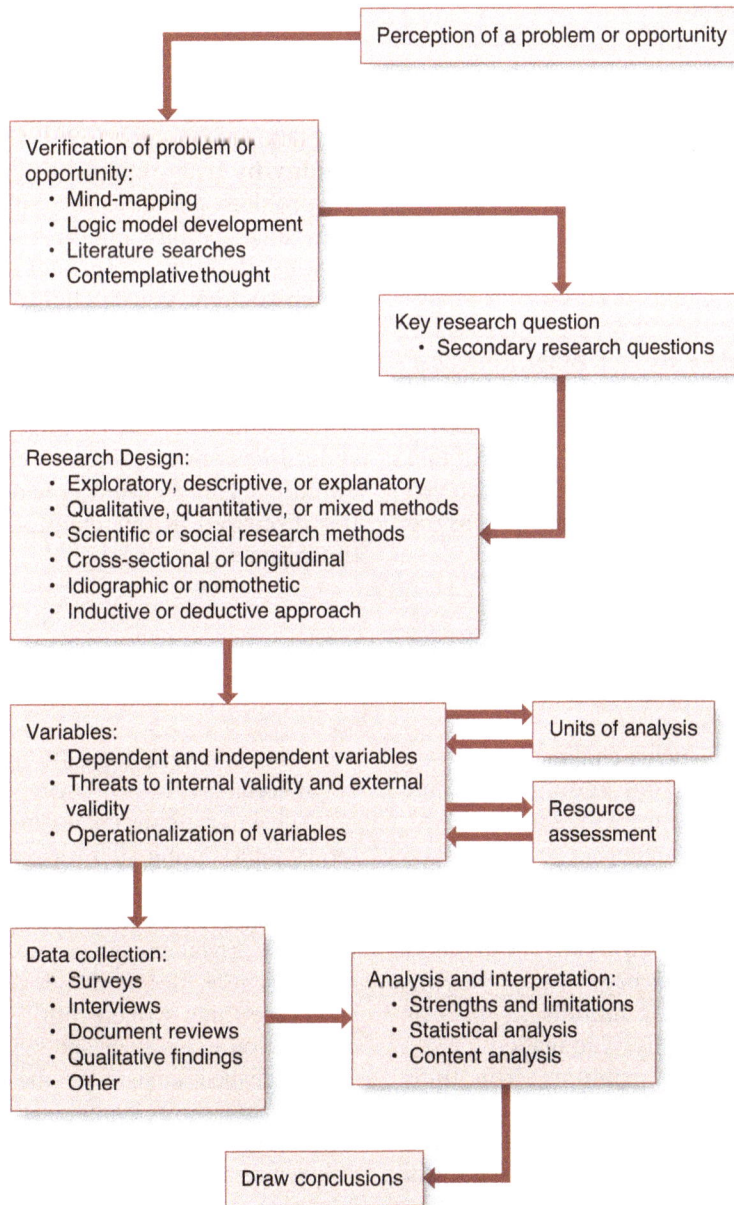

FIGURE 3.10 ■ Applying the principles of research to the analytical approach.

CHAPTER REVIEW

Summary

When faced with significant problems, or even opportunities for growth, a structured, well-designed analytical approach is essential for effective problem resolution or the best course of action. To accomplish this, knowledge of the components necessary for analysis, in what order they should be performed, and how they relate to each other is critical. The EMS analyst must be familiar with all aspects of analysis in order to choose the best options for success. In addition, he must build a solid foundation for analysis—best achieved by using established research principles as the central process.

The analysis must be objective, have validity by truly representing the nature of the problem, and have reliability in its determinations. By knowing the limitations of the various analytical approaches and how to minimize them, you can help ensure that you will arrive at the best solution. The strengths of your analytical approaches will help to establish credibility in your strategies for resolution. The entire analytical process should be meticulous, well controlled, and unbiased. Having the knowledge and abilities discussed in this chapter will facilitate those goals.

WHAT WOULD YOU DO? Reflection

Being faced with such a challenge as determining whether or not adding units and personnel despite a shrinking budget is feasible is likely to be daunting to most folks. But having a firm understanding of the analytical process enables you to begin to formulate a strategy for how you will proceed in your analysis. You begin by employing mind maps and logic models to discern whether or not the perceived inadequacy of services is truly the problem. You then translate the problem into a question that can be investigated and that will resolve your problem. You design your analysis based on established research principles and choose your variables and units of analysis carefully. You give considerable thought to the process of operationalization and spend some time developing good data collection instruments. You establish a time line and resource allocation budget and begin collecting information.

The information comes to you in many forms: interviewing staff, surveying the community, reviewing run documents, examining performance measures, gathering data on run statistics, projecting expenses and assessing net present values, and ultimately conducting a case study. Armed with all of this information, you begin your analysis. You employ some statistical analysis on the run data and content analysis on the qualitative reports. By integrating this information, you've arrived at a reasonable conclusion and can make an informed decision about how you should proceed. You've determined that you can exceed the breakeven point of costs in the first eight months and will likely have the support of the community and staff. You now feel confident in your decision to move forward with the plan.

Review Questions

1. How would you craft a key research question if you were faced with the challenge of analyzing the statement "Out-of-service times at the hospital are too long"?

2. Which research designs would be best suited to investigate lengthy out-of-service times at the hospital?

3. If you wanted to follow new employees on their endotracheal intubation performances for the year and compare them to the seasoned paramedics, what study type would be best?

4. How does the experimental design differ from the quasi-experimental design?

5. What are common examples of how social research is often conducted?

6. What are some of the advantages and limitations to longitudinal research over cross-sectional research?

7. If you were to examine prehospital mortality outcomes for cardiac arrest in the past 10 years and compare them to the present year performances, how would you categorize this type of study?

8. How does idiographic explanatory theory differ from nomothetic explanatory theory?

9. If you were to study the reasons that cause early burnout in the careers of paramedics, and looked at years of experience, age, level of training, average call volume per year, acuity and nature of calls, and organizational structure, which of these variables would likely be the dependent variable?

10. If you were studying paramedics in your agency to determine why their performances in endotracheal intubation are so varied and in doing so considered their age, number of intubation attempts annually, hours of education attained, and competency examination scores as independent variables, but discovered that years of experience was also a factor after the study, from what threat to variable selection does your study suffer?

11. In your study of endotracheal intubation performances, what would likely be the method of operationalization for the variable "competency examination scores"?

12. If one were to consider the belief that more education means improved patient outcomes, what investigative theory would you be employing?

13. To collect information on how much importance practicing EMS providers place on having health care benefits as part of their compensation package, you decide to conduct a survey asking respondents to rank their estimation from 1 to 5 in value. What features would be important in this collection instrument design, and how could you interpret the results?

14. In conducting person-to-person interviews, what important considerations must be kept in mind?

15. In your study to examine comparative performances among paramedics, advanced EMTs, and EMTs, you interview each provider category to seek insight into their perspective on their level of credential. What validity threat exists with this approach?

16. If you discover in your study of comparative performances among EMS providers that your study subject number is too large and you need help to conduct the interviews, with what internal validity threat should you be concerned?

17. If a study were to be conducted within a specific geographic region to determine provider competency in some select skill or set of skills, what limitation would that study have in terms of interpretation and applicability to the profession?

18. When conducting content analysis from transcribed interviews, you note the frequency of the occurrence of a particular word or phrase in all of the interviews. What is this form of content known as?

19. Statistical analysis has its basis in what foundational concepts?

20. Once you have completed your study based on the fundamental research principles, what additional steps should you consider before finalizing an analytical report?

References

Babbie, E. *The Practice of Social Research,* 13th ed.. (2013). Independence, KY: Wadsworth-Cengage Publishing.

Babbie, E. *The Basics of Social Research,* 5th ed. (2011). Independence, KY: Wadsworth-Cengage Publishing.

Campbell, D. T., and J. C. Stanley. (1963). *Experimental and Quasi-experimental Designs for Research.* Boston: Houghton Mifflin, 1963.

Creswell, J. W. (2009). *Research Design: Qualitative, Quantitative, and Mixed Methods Approaches,* 3rd ed. Thousand Oaks, CA: Sage Publications.

Greene, M., and D. Wright D. (2012). "2011 Salary & Workplace Survey," *JEMS 36*(10), pp. 42–.49

Framingham Heart Study. (2013). (See the organization website.)

IBM-SPSS Statistics, 200 W. Madison Street, Chicago, Illinois 60606. (See the organization website.)

Mason, J. (2002). *Qualitative Researching,* 2nd ed. Thousand Oaks, CA: Sage Publications.

SAS, SAS Institute, 100 SAS Campus Drive, Cary, Indiana 27513-2414. (See the organization website.)

Shadish, W. R., T. D. Cook, and D. T. Campbell. (2002). *Experimental and Quasi-experimental Designs for Generalized Causal Inference,* 2nd ed. Boston: Houghton-Mifflin.

Stata, StataCorp LP, 4905 Lakeway Drive, College Station, Texas 77845-4512. (See the organization website.)

Yin, R. K. *Case Study Research: Design and Methods,* 3rd ed. (2003). Thousand Oaks, CA: Sage Publications.

Key Terms

attrition effects A form of internal validity threat whereby subject withdraw or fall-out from the study occurs before the study ends, causing erroneous outcomes.

causality Creating an effect; being responsible for changing or creating a variable; a foundational component of statistical analysis.

coding A process of recording or denoting a value in the qualitative assessment of a document or transcription; transferring raw data into standardized forms for analysis.

cohort study A longitudinal study whereby the study group has some commonality or bond characteristic among the subjects.

concurrent research Research that is conducted at the same time as other research or during research design development; if qualitative and quantitative research are being conducted simultaneously (mixed methods), they are concurrent (if conducted serially, they are sequential).

confounding effects When the value of one (typically unknown) independent variable affects the value of another independent variable; when an extraneous, unknown variable covaries with another variable of interest.

content analysis An analytical process for the written word whereby concepts or repeating themes are identified and coded for later analysis.

continuous variable A numerical variable that has the potential for progressive value change, such as age.

correlation When one variable influences another variable with change; a criterion for proper variable selection whereby the chosen (independent) variable influences the dependent variable when change comes about.

data collection instrument Any device or construct that enables data collection; the most common forms are surveys, questionnaires, or tick forms.

deductive approach A theoretical structure of inquiry whereby a general concept, belief, or theory is used to guide the research and detailed factors are analyzed to determine if they support the overall theory or belief; from the general to the particulars.

dependent variable The central variable of interest in the study; the variable that answers the key research question; the variable that is *dependent* on the other, independent variables to exist or vary in value.

empirical process A process of formal analysis that abides by rules of structure and procedure to render valid and reliable data.

experimental design A form of quantitative research that allows randomization of subjects or interventions to study groups.

experimenter bias A threat to internal validity whereby the researcher (tester) conducting the data collection introduces selection bias into the study by behaving differently for some subjects or data elements than for others.

external validity Also known as generalization; having the quality of being able to apply the findings of the study from the select study population group to other, similar groups outside of the study; universal application of conclusions.

focus group interviews A form of qualitative inquiry that involves the researcher gathering interview data from groups of individuals simultaneously; typically, the individuals have some common link or association (e.g., members of a group, the general public, groups of co-workers, etc.).

Hawthorne effect An alteration in the subjects' behavior secondary to knowing that they are being assessed or tested; discovered at a production plant Illinois (Hawthorne Plant) and described by Elton Mayo.

history effects Events or behavioral changes that occur to subjects throughout the duration of the study that may affect the outcome under study.

idiographic explanation An investigative study approach to explanation whereby an exhaustive assessment of all of the possible causes of an event or phenomenon is conducted.

independent variable A variable in a study that is presumed to cause or alter the value of the dependent variable; variables of interest that are the subject of data collection in a study.

inductive approach A study approach whereby pieces of information are gathered through data collection into aggregate form to create a theory or central belief that offers explanation in the study; going from the particulars to the general.

Institutional Review Board A committee at universities and colleges comprised of profes-

sionals who oversee studies on human subjects to protect their rights and enforce medical ethics.

internal validity The quest of quantitative (and qualitative) research to ensure that the study design provides an explanation of causality between the independent and dependent variables.

key research question The guiding interrogative principle behind the study; the problem for which a solution is being sought in a general question format.

latent content In content analysis, discerning the underlying meaning for words or phrases intended by the interviewee; a subjective interpretation of the interviewee's meanings in statements.

Likert scale A scale format used in surveys and similar data collection instruments that provides the respondent with the option of indicating a valued response, typically on a numerical scale.

manifest content In content analysis, the obvious and declared meaning of statements from the interviewee taken for their face value, typically through a summation of occurrences in the interview.

maturation effects The consequences of when subjects in a study undergo natural changes that would occur otherwise in the study that may influence the study's outcome through threats of internal validity.

mixed methods design A research design that incorporates both quantitative as well as qualitative components; an approach that is becoming increasingly popular in its value and impact.

nomothetic explanation An investigative study approach to explanation whereby the most influential factors are examined closely, using probabilities and similar analyses for explanation.

nonspuriousness A criterion for variable selection that specifies that the variable of interest has no other outside factors of influence on the outcome variable; the relationship between the independent variable and dependent variable is uncorrupted.

operationalization The method or process to be employed in measuring the values of the variables of interest; to make the variable contributory in the study.

panel study A longitudinal study whereby the study group is followed over a period of time with a focus on some characteristic common to each of them; they may be disparate otherwise and not of a common group; similar to a cohort study.

prospective research A form of longitudinal research that looks to the future for data collection and results; these studies are very effective as the design is preliminarily determined and all controls can be put into place before the study begins.

qualitative design A fundamental research design that studies events or phenomenon of a nonnumerical nature, typically of a behavioral or communication nature, and attempts to disclose underlying meanings and patterns of relationships.

quantitative design A fundamental research design that studies events or phenomena of a numerical nature, typically through observations, interventions, precise measurements, and statistical probability predictions to disclose underlying relationships of causality.

quasi-experimental design Quantitative research that is similar to experimental design, but without the advantage of randomization of subjects or interventions.

retrospective research A form of longitudinal research that looks into the past for information and data collection; these studies are convenient as the data already exist, but somewhat less effective as the controls cannot be put into place before the study begins.

secondary research question Research questions borne from the identified problem that modify or supplement the key research question; secondary research questions often seek additional information for clarification of the key research question.

selection bias A common threat of internal validity whereby choosing subject participation or exposing subjects to interventions is nonrandomized and often under some conscious or unconscious bias; this type of bias may influence outcomes.

self-reporting bias A type of internal validity threat that results from the subject providing information directly under the full awareness of the purpose; as it is human nature to depict oneself in the "best light," there may be some embellishment of data.

telephonic survey A method of conducting a survey through the means of contacting the respondent via telephone; the interviewer follows a predetermined script and records the interviewee's responses.

testing effects A threat to internal validity caused by subjects being tested repeatedly; also a form of threat that results from the subject being aware of the testing process (*see* Hawthorne effect).

time order A criterion for variable selection that specifies that the effects resulting from the variable of interest has an impact on the dependent variable, and, so, must precede the independent variable in time.

trend study A form of longitudinal research whereby the study population possesses some characteristic of study interest, but otherwise lacks any commonality.

typology A systematic classification of varying forms of a subject, concept, or categories based on similar characteristics; a classification or categorization.

units of analysis An important element in study design that specifies the what or whom being studied.

variables A known or unknown element in an equation that is representative of a set of attributes unique to that element.

Financial Analysis

4 CHAPTER

Objectives

After reading this chapter, the student should be able to:

4.1 Relate the importance of the basics of financial analysis in the overall analysis approach and the relevance of financial statements.

4.2 Describe the features and components of the balance sheet, how each is derived, and how they relate to each other.

4.3 Describe the features and components of the income statement, how each is derived, and how they relate to each other.

4.4 Describe the features and components of the cash flow statement, how each is derived, how they relate to each other, what the various sources of cash may be, and how cash is recorded.

4.5 Demonstrate an understanding of the importance of footnotes to financial statements and the Generally Accepted Accounting Principles.

4.6 Describe the compositional elements of the more common financial ratios, their benefits, limitations, interrelationships, and contributions toward the analytical approach.

4.7 Describe the basic process, theoretical foundation, and benefits and limitations of a breakeven analysis in financial assessment.

4.8 Describe the nature and benefits of pro forma statements and their contribution to financial analysis.

4.9 Describe the concept of the time value of money and relate those principles to financial analysis.

4.10 Demonstrate an understanding of how the financial analytical processes contribute to the overall analytical approach for EMS.

Key Terms

accelerated
  depreciation
accounts payable
accrued expenses
accumulated
  depreciation
asset turnover ratio
assets
balance sheet
breakeven analysis
breakeven point
capital stock
cash disbursements
cash flow statement
cash receipts
costs of services
current assets
current debt
current liabilities
current ratios
debt ratio

discounting future
  value
double-declining
  balance
  depreciation
EBIT
ending cash balance
equity
fixed asset purchases
fixed assets
fixed costs
GAAP
general and
  administrative
  expenses
gross margin
gross profit
incidental services
income from
  operations
income statement

income taxes payable
interest coverage
interest on income
leverage
leverage ratios
liabilities
liquidity
liquidity ratios
long-term debt
long-term liabilities
net borrowings
net current assets
net income
net sales (or net
  services)
net worth
non-cash transactions
operating expenses
operating leverage
present value
pro forma statements

profit margin
profitability ratios
quick ratio
retained earnings
return on assets
return on services
revenues
shareholder's equity
straight-line
  depreciation
sum-of-years
  depreciation
time value of money
total assets
total costs
unit hour utilization
  analysis (UHUA)
variable costs
working capital

WHAT WOULD YOU DO?

You are the operations director for a medium-size EMS system in a fairly rural community. The call volume has steadily grown proportionately with the population growth of your coverage area. Your crews are insisting that there is a need for an additional advanced life support unit to supplement the ambulances and crews that you already have. There is plenty of evidence that they are right—crews are being forced to return to service much more quickly, and average response times are getting longer due to the increased volume of calls.

1. Can your organization afford a new, fully equipped ambulance? You certainly don't have money to meet the price in the service's bank account. Will the bank be willing to loan you the money?

2. How financially efficient has your organization been?

3. With the current rate of growth, will you be able to sustain this level of demand much longer?

4. How can you project operational income for the next year, 3 years, or 5 years?

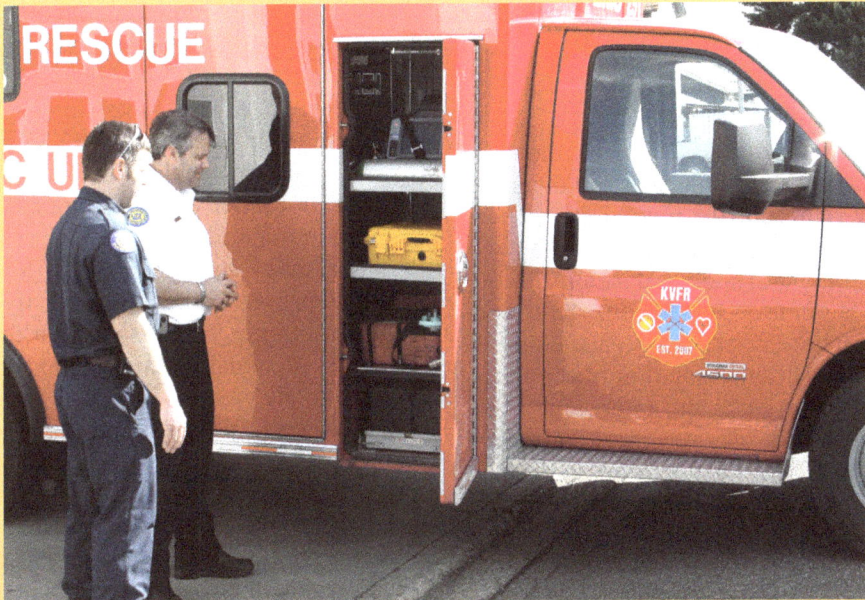

FIGURE 4.1 ■ The operations director considers a new ambulance.

■ INTRODUCTION

In virtually every instance of analysis, there is a need to know what the cost of the problem will be, or what will likely be the cost of fixing the problem, or venturing into this new opportunity. Moreover, if an organization is contemplating an opportunity for growth or perhaps investing in a costly solution to a significant problem, it is imperative that a clear understanding of the organization's solvency and economic status be determined.

In essence, financial analysis is often a critical component of every analytical approach. For this reason, we will explore the realm of the financial analyst with the intent of learning the basic essentials, techniques of analysis, and how to interpret financial indicators.

Often when one is presented with a challenge to discern the financial status of an organization or the long-term cost of a project, the initial response is to seek out a financial expert as we may consider these matters outside of our realm of understanding. Although this may be necessary for complex or unusually large projects, that may not always be the case for most analytical endeavors. Many financial analyses can be carried out by the EMS manager or administrator with only a better understanding of the principles of financial analysis. Having that knowledge will go a long way to better understanding most analytical situations, avoiding wrong decisions, and incurring unnecessary costs.

BASICS OF FINANCIAL ANALYSIS—

For many organizations, financial data are often the driving force in decision making and frequently represent the pivotal component regarding which direction a decision may go. The decision to move forward on a project or endeavor is often dependent on what financial gain can be realized. Costly endeavors will most often result in dissolution of the initiative. This underscores the importance that financial analysis plays in most important decisions and its critical role in analysis of EMS systems and organizations. Therefore, having a thorough understanding of financial analysis is essential, and there is no better place to begin than with the basics.

When one considers financial matters, we often think about account statements or summary reports on fiscal information. This approach is fine, but we need to take it one step further: We need to examine official financial statements. Understanding what financial statements are, what different types exist, how each one provides different information, and how to integrate the information gathered from all of them will prove to be very valuable.

FINANCIAL STATEMENTS————

Let's begin by identifying the most commonly used financial statements: the **balance sheet**, the **income statement**, and the **cash flow statement**. Each of these has value in and of itself, but together they provide a clear perspective into an organization's financial status, and to some degree, performance. Typically, the first financial statement to examine is the balance sheet.

BALANCE SHEET

The balance sheet represents the financial status of an organization at a moment in time—a "financial snapshot." It demonstrates, and compares, what the organization owns or has at that moment in time (**assets**), what it owes to other entities (**liabilities**), and what the organization's **net worth** is (**equity**). Each of these components should be found on any balance sheet, but *remember*—the balance sheet represents that status only at that moment in time. This is similar in concept to the cross-sectional research design that looks at data at one moment in time.

Figure 4.2 provides an example of the components of a simple balance sheet. As you can see, each category in the balance sheet has many subcomponents that represent that category. For example, Assets consists of the amount of cash on hand, the amount of money to be received within a specific time frame that is reasonably assured, any inventory of value, and **fixed assets** (property, plant, and equipment or PP&E). Although these terms and designations are generic and can apply to any organization, for clarity and understanding, we will use examples that apply to EMS to illustrate these features.

Assets

As mentioned, assets represent what the organization owns. It is typically denoted as either **current assets** or fixed assets. Current assets, by definition, are those assets that are expected to be converted into cash within the next year. They are often referred to as the

---

Balance Sheet Components

Current Date

Assets	**Liabilities and Equity**
Cash	Accounts Payable
Accounts Receivable	Accrued Expenses
Inventory	Current Debt (annual)
Prepaid Expenses	Income Tax (annual)
Current Assets Total	Current Liabilities Total
Other Assets	Long-term Debt
Fixed Assets at Cost	Capital Stock
Accumulated Depreciation	Retained Earnings
Net Fixed Assets	Shareholder's Equity
Total Assets	Total Liabilities & Equity

FIGURE 4.2 Components of a simple balance sheet.

most liquid. **Liquidity** refers to the ability to convert an asset into cash quickly. Obviously, the most liquid asset is cash itself! In general, assets are listed on the balance sheet in order from the most liquid to the least liquid. This helps in quickly approximating how much cash-on-hand an organization can have with one glance at the balance sheet.

Under current assets on the balance sheet, you should expect to find listed cash, accounts receivable, inventory, and prepaid expenses. Cash simply is the amount of actual cash the organization has on hand. Accounts receivable are those monetary amounts that are currently owed the organization. In EMS, this may very well be the money billed for services already rendered in which payment is reasonably expected. In general, inventory is not applicable to EMS organizations since a product is not produced but, rather, a service is provided. If EMS were in the business of producing items (let's say first-aid kits), then inventory would be the number of products (first-aid kits) that are on the shelf and not yet distributed. However, soft supplies and medi-

cal items may be stocked in EMS systems, in which case they could be included as inventory for the purposes of asset assessment. Prepaid expenses are services or products to be used by the organization (we'll use uniform cleaning as the example) that have not yet been expended. Some EMS agencies will pay (under contract) to have the crew's uniforms laundered by an outside service on a quarterly or annual basis, even though the service has not yet been rendered. The uniforms yet to be laundered (in the future) represent prepaid services and are eligible as current assets.

In addition to current assets, a balance sheet may also include fixed assets. These are assets that are less likely to be converted into cash (less liquidity) and are often comprised of plant, property, and equipment. In EMS, these would consist of the building, any satellite stations, the property owned by the organization, and all of the durable equipment (ambulances, aid cars, stretchers, monitor/defibrillators office equipment, etc.). In many organizations, fixed assets represent the largest valued assets a company owns. In addition, as we know, *physical plants* (a financial term that refers to buildings and offices), property, and durable equipment will depreciate over time. For this reason, balance sheets will often list both the value of the fixed asset at the time of acquisition (known as the fixed asset at cost) and the depreciated value of the fixed asset (known as the net fixed asset). The amount the asset is depreciated is often listed as **accumulated depreciation**. The actual depreciation is recorded in a separate financial statement known as the income statement (see discussion later in this chapter). It is important to note that some assets do not depreciate but, rather, *appreciate* over time. This, too, is reflected in the balance sheet.

Some balance sheets may also list other assets. This represents assets that are somewhat intangible and difficult to fit into the other asset categories. If an EMS agency has a well-known name in the trade industry, perhaps that name has some associated value. If so, it deserves to be valued in the asset category.

Traditional balance sheets will then sum the current assets to the fixed assets to report the **total assets**. Total assets then represent the entire value owned by the company. It is used in the calculation of net value (see below).

Liabilities

Like assets, liabilities can be categorized. Most balance sheets list liabilities as **current liabilities**, **long-term liabilities** (or debt), or **shareholder's equity**. Collectively, the liabilities side of the balance sheet represents the economic obligations the organization has to its creditors, agents, or employees.

Current liabilities are comprised of expenses that must be paid within 1 year. Often, the money used to pay the current liabilities come from the current assets category. Current liabilities often consist of **accounts payable**, **accrued expenses**, and **current debt**. Accounts payable are those expenses owed

vendors for services rendered or products provided, often through a credit arrangement. If an EMS agency purchased soft supplies (disposable goods) from a particular vendor, then the amount owed for those supplies would fall under accounts payable. In this particular instance, if the supplies were already received, then the value of those items (supply assets) will exactly equal the accounts payable amount for those items (less the taxes or other incidental costs).

Accrued expenses are similar to accounts payable, but they differ in to whom the debt is owed. In the previous example, the accounts payable was monies owed a vendor for soft supplies; for accrued expenses, the owed amount would be to employees, banks for interest, or similar forms of payment. So, salaries earned by paid employees are not categorized under accounts payable, but under accrued expenses instead.

Current debt is simply those expenses that are owed and to be paid within 1 year. It can even represent the annual debt of a multi-year debt obligation. Annual income tax will fall under current debt, as will any other annual tax liability as long as its period is less than 1 year. Income tax expenses are often listed separately as **income taxes payable** to distinguish them from other current liabilities.

If the debt obligation is longer than 1 year, it is termed **long-term debt**, which is also a component of the liabilities section. Basically, long-term debt is any loan to the organization that has a life of more than 12 months. The most common examples are equity loans, mortgages, and long-term rental agreements.

Shareholder's Equity

Even though shareholder's equity is listed separately in a balance sheet, it represents a somewhat unusual form of debt to an organization. It is the debt owed the shareholders after the expenses of the liabilities are deducted from all of the assets of the organization. What is left over (some would say "profit") belongs to the owners of the organization or shareholders. Clearly, this concept implies either a privately owned company or a publicly traded organization. However, the organization may be neither, but the application of the concept remains the same. This is because shareholder's equity means the same as net worth. So, even if the organization is not privately owned or publicly traded, when you deduct the liabilities from the assets, what remains is the organization's net worth. What happens if the liabilities exceed the assets? Then you have a situation in which the net worth is negative or "upside down" in its value. This has, unfortunately, become a well-known principle resulting from the recent economic collapse of the housing market and increasing interest rates of the mortgage companies.

Shareholder's equity can also be categorized. It is typically declared as either **capital stock** (in a stock-invested company) or **retained earnings** (the money not paid-out in dividends). Keep in mind that shareholder's equity is the same as net worth. That means that in organizations which are not privately owned or publicly traded, the difference between the assets and liabilities (net worth) is simply the amount left over (and if assets exceed liabilities, then it *is* profit).

For illustrative purposes, a fabricated, simple balance sheet is provided in Figure 4.3. Consider the information contained in this example for the principles and concepts mentioned earlier and apply the actual numbers to the formulae below.

Using the Balance Sheet Information

If you were to add up all of the liabilities (current and long-term debt) and combine that with the shareholder's equity amount (which, once again, could be retained earnings or net

WeCare EMS End-of-Year Balance Sheet	
Assets	
Cash and cash equivalents	$89,000
Accounts receivable	179,000
CPR training and other accounts receivable (net)	12,000
Supplies inventory	45,780
Prepaids and other current assets	16,417
Current deferred assets	12,473
Property, plant, and equipment (net)	436,014
Intangible assets	66,789
Insurance collateral	158,790
Other long-term assets	29,678
Capital grant	200,328
Goodwill	72,000
Total Assets: $1,318,269	
Liabilities	
Accounts payable	$65,172
Accrued liabilities	231,631
Current portion of long-term debt	4,159
Income taxes	52
Long-term notes payable	475,616
Insurance reserves and other long-term liabilities	155,599
Capital stock	212,361
Retained earnings	173,679
Total Liabilities: $1,318,269	

FIGURE 4.3 ■ Sample balance sheet.

worth) and subtract that from all of the assets (current and fixed), you should come up with a zero balance. All of the assets should equal the sum of all of the liabilities plus the shareholder's equity. Or, in equation form:

Assets − Liabilities + Shareholder's Equity = Zero

A variation of this equation can be quite useful. Consider what you would have if you removed the shareholder's equity from the left side of the equation. For example:

$$\text{Assets} - \text{Liabilities} = ?$$

The answer is net worth. So, simply looking at a balance sheet and examining the total assets and total liabilities, you can quickly determine an organization's net worth.

From another perspective, let's examine portions of the balance sheet components, specifically, the current assets and current liabilities. If you think about this, the current assets are those that are most liquid and the current liabilities are those that the organization is obliged to pay within the year, and then you may realize the value of this relationship. Let's look at it in the formula format:

Current Assets − Current Liabilities
= **Working Capital**

You now have a new measure from the balance sheet: working capital. This represents what the organization has to work with in the short term (within 1 year). It is sometimes referred to as **net current assets** (since it is the current assets "net" the current liabilities). What is the value of this parameter? Well, organizations that have a lot of working capital are able to satisfy its 1-year debt obligations easily— some would say this is a well-run organization. However, what purpose is that money serving as working capital? Others would argue that such an organization with a large amount of working capital is a poorly run organization because it is squandering money that could be invested. As you can see, it depends on one's perspective and the purpose of the organization.

There are many other uses of the balance sheet and its information. These additional uses are beyond the scope of this chapter and interested readers are encouraged to explore texts specific to financial analysis. You can probably already see the value of looking at the balance sheet of an organization. Let's examine more financial statements.

INCOME STATEMENT

Of the financial statements, the balance sheet and the income statement are the most often used and probably the most revealing of an organization's financial status. The income statement reveals the organization's cash movements and can indicate its profitability. Where the balance sheet reports the financial status of an organization at a moment in time, the income statement indicates the financial activities over a period of time (often a month or quarter, or even a year). In general, it reveals what was sold or what services were rendered in that period, what it cost to produce that product or service, and what monies remained as income. The income statement says nothing about what the organization has in total, just what was reported for that period of time.

So, in formula format, the income statement can be summarized as:

Revenue from Sales (Services) − Operating Costs & Expenses = Income

We again relate these concepts in an EMS context. Typically, an income statement is depicted as sales, but EMS doesn't provide product; it provides service, so we'll substitute "sales" with "services."

Revenues

When considering income statements, since we are examining revenue versus expenses, we must separate the inputs into either **revenues** or expenses. Revenue often has many contributing components, but in an income statement, they are organized according to the delivery of services and other sources of income. So, in our example, we will categorize the first part of the income statement as revenue from services and then determine our **gross profit** by deducting our cost of delivery of services. Figure 4.4 illustrates that level of organization within an income statement.

Income Statement	How Derived
Income Statement	**How Derived**
Period from month/day/year to month/day/year	
A Net Services	$$$
B Cost of Services	$$$
Gross Profit:	A − B
C Cost of Incidental Services	$$$
D Marketing Expenses	$$$
E General and Administrative Expenses	$$$
Operating Expenses:	C + D + E
F Income from Operations	(A − B) − (C + D + E)
G Interest on Income	$$$
H Income Tax Expense	$$$
Net Income:	(A − B) − (C + D + E) + G − H

FIGURE 4.4   Components of an income statement.

Net Sales (or Services). The term **net services** more aptly captures what an EMS agency delivers: services. So, we'll replace **net sales** with net services. Services are the revenues generated by the delivery of services in the given time period. It is important to recognize that this must represent services already delivered and not any anticipated services.

Costs of Services. Now, to determine the gross profit for the period, we must first determine what was the cost incurred to deliver those services. This is listed in the first part of the income statement as illustrated in Figure 4.4. Here, we are listing what expenditures were necessary *strictly* to deliver the services during that period, whether it was fuel for ambulances, payroll for employees, costs of soft supplies, cost of medical materials depleted (like pharmaceutical items), expended portions of oxygen, and other routinely expended materials or expenses. It is important to constrain these **costs of services** to *strictly* those costs associated with directly

delivering the service. See the sidebar regarding an important difference between cost and expenses.

Side Bar

A Few Words about Costs and Expenses

In general, costs are those expenditures necessary to deliver the services directly. Examples include the cost of supplies, drugs, salaries of the crew, gasoline for the ambulance, intravenous solution, soft supplies, and paperwork.

By comparison, expenses are those expenditures that fall outside of the direct delivery of services, such as administrative or clerical support salaries, insurance premiums, maintenance expenses, depreciation of capital goods, and educational costs.

Knowing the subtle distinction between costs and expenses will help a lot in understanding how the income statement and the balance sheet work together.

As may be obvious at this point, having a clear understanding of the costs associated with delivery of services is very important in the overall financial picture and in any organizational analysis.

Gross Profit. At this point, if we were to take all of the revenues generated during this time period (net services) and deduct the associated costs to deliver those services, we would end up with our gross profit—the amount of revenue realized from the "sale" of services, less the costs to deliver those services. Gross profit is sometimes referred to as **gross margin**.

Expenses

Please review the clarification of costs and expenses in the sidebar feature. In this portion of the income statement, the expenses of the organization are listed. Here, we will examine other service expenses, the expense for marketing, and **general and administrative expenses**.

Incidental Services. If the service delivered by the EMS agency is not directly related to its primary mission or purpose, then it could be considered an incidental service. These services still have costs associated with them. For example, if your agency is requested to stand by at sporting events or fires, even though no medical services may be actually provided, there is an expense associated with being there. These are the incidental service expenses. They may include conducting blood pressure screenings, providing public education, conducting a CPR class, or participating in a community event or meeting. Many organizations consider such activities as the cost of doing business. However, if they are not accounted for in your financial statements, then (from a financial perspective) they do not exist. Often, these **incidental services** bring great value to the organization and may also create some significant expense.

Marketing. Most EMS agencies want to improve their public image and enhance their services, whether it be the coverage area or the scope of services to be delivered. Any effort to market the organization has an associated cost that must be recorded. Creating, generating, and distributing brochures about your organization, putting ads in the local paper or radio station, and participating in public promotion of your agency are examples of marketing efforts. The expenses tied to these activities should be recorded in the income statement as well.

General and Administrative Expenses. This is likely to be your greatest indirect cost of delivering services. It largely consists of everything else other than direct service delivery costs, such as clerical and office staff expenses, accounting expenses, copier contracts, billing services, health benefit expenses, accreditation expenses, and professional fees. Some of these expenses are assessed over the period of a year. If the income statement is for a period less than a year, then the administrative and general expenses are prorated accordingly to reflect the period of time of the income statement.

Operating Expenses

The **operating expenses** are those expenditures that the organization dispenses in the course of the delivery of services in order to generate revenue. It is a collective concept that is represented by the incidental service expenses, the marketing expenses, and the general and administrative expenses. It is derived simply by adding those components together, and it is listed in the income statement on a separate line. See Figure 4.4 for illustration.

Income from Operations

When considering all of the costs associated with the delivery of services (incidental services, marketing, and general and administrative expenses) and deducting that from the gross profit that was earned by its delivery, what remains is the **income from operations**. This is the financial benefit the organization derives from doing business. There also exists income earned from non-operating activities, such as investment, sale of property, or stock growth, but these would be recorded elsewhere in the income statement.

Interest on Income

Recall that there also are expenses not associated with the delivery of service. These expenses, such as interest on a loan or insurance premiums, would be recorded under general and administrative expenses. However, interest that is *earned* on the income already received, such as in an interest-earning account or certificate of deposit, is traditionally recorded under **interest on income**.

Income Taxes

The expenses of taxes paid on income is logged on the income statement as income taxes. If the income statement is for a period less than 1 year, then the amount under income taxes is prorated to reflect that portion of taxes to be paid out.

Net Income

The line of the income statement labeled as **net income** represents the overall income the organization realizes after all income from operations is added to the interest income and operating expenses and expenses from taxation are deducted. This is what most people refer to as "the bottom line" in financial parlance. It is, in fact, located on the bottom line of the income statement and reveals the organization's overall income for the period designated in the income statement.

Using Income Statement Information

The income statement provides the analyst with information related to the organization's current revenues versus expenses. It is reflective of the agency's efficiency at making a profit. However, it says nothing about how much money the company has or how much profit (or loss) the organization has experienced beyond the period of interest in the income statement. As is often the case with any investigation, to obtain a clear, overall picture, one must examine multiple aspects of the situation.

Examining what the organization currently possesses in assets and expenditures and how it receives revenue and expends money are the stories told by the organization's balance sheet and income statement. The two are closely linked and interdependent. When gross profit falls for a period of time, expenses will sometimes accumulate and the organization's assets will be reduced to offset the additionally incurred expenses. Also, the income statement reflects, for the period, what actions were taken by the organization to increase assets and even decrease liabilities. The two financial statements tell a lot about an organization's financial health.

However, in the contribution of financial analysis toward the analytical approach, it is important to consider all of the financial statements. Even though the balance sheet and the income statement are the most popular and informative, we must still consider the value of the cash flow statement. We will examine that statement next.

CASH FLOW STATEMENT

The cash flow statement basically reveals how the organization obtains its cash and where the cash goes—it tracks the "flow of cash" over a period of time. Think of what transactions the organization undergoes at any given time and you can appreciate what the statement of cash flows demonstrates.

For example, when the EMS agency receives payments for services rendered, this increases the amount of cash the agency has. When it pays salaries to its workers, the amount of cash is then reduced. This fluctuation of money in and out of the organization represents the cash flow. It can only occur with cash exchanges (or similar transactions like credit account debits or checking account credits) that actually affect the amount of money in the organization's accounts. There are other exchanges that are considered **non-cash transactions**.

These events do not directly affect the amount of cash or money in the organization's accounts when they occur. Examples of non-cash transactions would be the actual delivery of EMS service, or the receipt of soft supplies to stock the ambulance, or the delivery of office products. These occurrences will eventually result in some cash flow (revenue receipt, payment of a vendor, etc.), but at the time of occurrence, they do not and therefore are termed non-cash transactions. Non-cash transactions will impact the balance sheet and the income statement but not the cash flow statement.

So, the cash flow statement is all about the cash and whether it's increasing or decreasing over a period of time. It is a good measure of the organization's liquidity. Since it depicts cash flow over a period of time, it reveals the amount of cash at the start of the period, the amount of cash received in that period, the amount of cash spent in that period, and, therefore, the amount of cash on hand at the end of that period. An example of the cash flow statement elements is illustrated in Figure 4.5.

When you consider what happens to generate the cash flow statement, you may realize that the cash flow statement is nothing more than the comparison of a balance sheet at the beginning of the period to a balance sheet at the end of the period using some elements from the income statement to illustrate the nature of those monetary changes. The cash flow statement helps to explain the changes between two consecutive balance sheets. So, in effect, the concepts of two of the financial statements (the balance sheet and the income statement) can be integrated to form a dynamic picture of money movement through the development of the cash flow statement. It is important to note that the cash flow statement is not solely derived from these two other financial statements, but rather that they contribute, in concept, to the development of the cash flow statement. The nature of

Cash Flow Statement	How Derived
Period from month/day/year to month/day/year	
A Beginning Cash Balance	$$$
B Cash Receipts	$$$
C Cash Disbursements (outlays)	$$$
Cash From Operations:	B − C
D Fixed Asset Purchases	$$$
E Net Borrowings	$$$
F Income Taxes Paid	$$$
G Sales of Stock	$$$
Ending Cash Balance:	A + (B − C) − D + E − F + G

FIGURE 4.5 ■ Components of a cash flow statement.

changes between two balance sheets in consecutive periods and data from the income statement during the same period can be revealed through the cash flow statement.

Generally, the cash flow statement reveals information of cash movement on three fronts: investments, operations, and financing. The investments are derived from the assets listed in the balance sheet, the cash flow from operations is derived from the income statement in income from operations or net income, and the financing component is the total liabilities or net worth, again from the balance sheet. In fact, many cash flow statements are organized to reflect these divisions, as illustrated in Figure 4.6.

The investments section is altered by the acquisition of assets, the sale of assets (termed disinvestments), and the effect of depreciation (more on that later). The operations portion is impacted by price, cost (variable and fixed), and volume (more on that later, too), whereas the financing section is determined by matters of debt, retained earnings, dividends, and paid interest.

Sources of Cash

Generally, when we think of cash flow in an organization, we think about the receipt (or payout) of money. But how is that money received? In the EMS industry, it is usually in the form of payment for services. We regard this source of money as money from operating activities. The movement of money can go both ways. In operating activities, we also need to purchase supplies and pay salaries to operate effectively. This would represent an *outflow* of cash.

Another source of cash is through investments. This could be an investment in mutual funds, stocks, rental of properties (as in renting a hall for an activity), or even borrowing money (it is a form of investment—you pay money over time for a large sum immediately).

Cash Flow Statement		
Year:	Year 1	Year 2
Operating Activities		
Net Earnings from Services (operations)	$$$	$$$
Net Cash on Hand	$$$	$$$
Accounts Receivable	$$$	$$$
Accounts Payable	$$$	$$$
Inventories, Capital Goods, Prepaid Expenses	$$$	$$$
Investing Activities		
Capital Expenditures	$$$	$$$
Assets (PP&E)	$$$	$$$
Acquisitions and Divestitures	$$$	$$$
Financing Activities		
Short-term debt	$$$	$$$
Long-term debt	$$$	$$$
Dividends	$$$	$$$
Interest (including net borrowings)	$$$	$$$
Ending Cash Balance:		

FIGURE 4.6   Cash flow statement using operating, investment, and financing activities.

At any rate, investment is a source of cash flow *into* the organization. However, it is also a means by which cash flows *out of* the organization—through interest rates and payments on principal.

Even purchasing sizable assets (a new ambulance, a new building, or some new equipment) is a cash flow concern. Even though it increases the assets category on the balance sheet, it still represents a cash outlay for the organization. Paying taxes is also a form of cash outflow.

Cash Receipts

It can then be realized that collecting payments from customers for services rendered is a primary form of cash flow *into* the organization. From the cash flow statement, these receipts will increase the amount of cash on hand for the organization. This impact is probably obvious. What may not be so obvious is that there is often a complementary impact on the other side of the balance sheet—the liabilities side. When payment is received for services, it increases the cash on hand (assets), but it equally decreases the current liabilities (accounts receivable) at the same time. Although we like to think of cash flow into the organization as profits, in financial analysis the two are distinctly different. Profits are listed in the income statement, whereas cash appears on the balance sheets and cash flow statements.

Cash Disbursements (outlays)

Whereas cash flow into the organization is termed **cash receipts**, cash disbursement is cash flow *out* of the organization. This typically occurs in the form of payments—payments for salaries, payments for goods received, payments on past loans, and so on. Clearly, **cash disbursements** lower the amount of cash on hand in the cash flow statement and reduce the assets in the balance sheet. On the other

hand, cash disbursements are necessary to acquire assets.

Cash from Operations

As mentioned, services rendered are the most common form of revenue generation in EMS. This is the cash from operations. It is represented on the cash flow statement by the activities of cash receipts and cash disbursements in the course of the organization's operations. Figure 4.5 illustrates that relationship, where cash disbursements are deducted from cash receipts to reveal the cash from operations. (Note: This is *not* added to cash on hand—that remains until the end of the cash flow statement.) Cash flow from operations provides the reader with a quick assessment of the amount of cash being generated during a designated period of operations.

Fixed Asset Purchases

A major form of cash disbursement is the acquisition of property, plant, and equipment. Sizable acquisitions such as these will reduce the cash assets significantly, but add to the capital assets of the organization. These are known as **fixed asset purchases** because they have little or no liquidity and often remain with the organization for some time. They are also not part of the operations disbursement of cash, but they are listed separately in the cash flow statement. Once again, disbursements of cash for the acquisition of fixed assets should be reflected in the balance sheet under fixed assets. This is another means of checks and balances in the financial operations of an organization.

Net Borrowings

When an organization borrows money from a lender, it acquires additional cash. This adds to the cash flow *into* the organization and is depicted on the cash flow statement. However, these loans must be paid back, usually with interest. Therefore, there is also a cash flow *out of* the organization for the purposes of paying back these preexisting loans. For this reason, we often report borrowings as "net" borrowings so as to indicate the result of cash flows in both directions. If the organization has gained more borrowed money than it paid out for previous loans, then the **net borrowings** will be positive. If the reverse is the case, then the net borrowings will be negative. A quick glance at the net borrowings on the cash flow statement gives a rough indication as to what degree of debt an organization might have at a given period of time. If the net borrowings line is negative, the organization is likely to have some long-term liabilities that should also be reflected in the balance sheet.

Income Taxes Paid

Each time an organization must pay out in income tax, that portion of its revenue must be recorded on the cash flow statement as income taxes paid. It should only represent the amount of taxes paid, not owed. Owed income tax will be paid in the future and will later appear on the cash flow statements of the future. Paying of income taxes represents a cash flow *out of* the organization for the period of time under review.

Sales of Stock

In traded organizations, the sale of common or preferred stock is a source of income that is reported on the cash flow statement as well as the income statement. In the cash flow statement, it is recorded on a separate line to indicate the amount of cash flow *into* the organization from the sale of capital stock in the given time period under review. The purchase of stock is an investment into the organization by the buyers and represents a level of confidence that the organization will perform better in the future and its value will consequently increase. It benefits the consumer by the purchase and the organization by the cash flow into the organization.

Ending Cash Balance

The **ending cash balance** is quite simply the transactional result of the amount of money the organization had at the beginning of the period, the amount of cash into and out of the organization during that period, and the amount of money that is now left over. By considering the first line of the cash flow statement, the beginning cash balance, and then adding and deducting each of the line items on the statement as listed above, the resulting amount is the ending cash balance for that period.

In a sense, the ending cash balance is a simple gauge of the organization's profitability during the period under examination. What must be kept in mind is that it does *not* represent the organization's financial performance overall, but merely the cash acquisitions (or outlays) during that time. For example, if the organization used a sizable amount of its cash on hand to purchase property or equipment, its cash on hand would decrease considerably. Yet, its asset values would increase proportionally. This action might indeed demonstrate marked successes in the organization, but the cash flow statement would suggest otherwise. This is, in part, the reason that we must always consider all financial statements of an organization when conducting an analysis.

SOME FINAL THOUGHTS ON FINANCIAL STATEMENTS

Financial statements are the blueprints of the organization's financial status. They reveal financial activities in many aspects of performance. As such, they must be considered with each other, as well as with additional information regarding the organization's status, performance, and vision. Much like a physical examination of a patient, we never place too much emphasis on one part of our assessment, but rather integrate our findings to create an overall picture.

It is also important to note that the financial statements have another vital element that we haven't discussed. That is the notes to financial statements. These appear as footnotes at the end of each financial statement. Their importance is based on the fact that these notes reveal many of the organization's financial practices, rules, explanations, reasons for certain decisions, and other supportive information. They help to clarify the information found on the financial statement.

In addition, it is important to note that although each organization may differ from others in its structure, type, purpose, size, and even growth, the manner in which its financial performance is reported is fundamentally the same. Organizations are bound to report financial data in accordance with Generally Accepted Accounting Principles, or **GAAP**, which represent a standardization of format, descriptors, and purposes of the financial statements. These are established by the Financial Accounting Standards Board (FASB) under the auspices of the U.S. Securities and Exchange Commission (SEC).

In summary, financial statements are critical to the financial analysis of any organization. It is important that we consider all financial statements and compare those findings to other sources of information. We should examine the balance sheet to learn of the organization's financial condition at a point in time and see the cumulative effect of previous decisions. We should examine the income statement to discover the revenues and expenses of the organization during a period of time. And, we should examine the cash flow statement to appreciate the dynamic nature in the changes of assets and liabilities of the organization and gain a perspective on

its cash flow activity. From this information, we can effectively conduct the necessary financial analysis of the organization to supplement our analytical approach to problem solving or decision making for opportunities for growth.

■ CONDUCTING THE FINANCIAL ANALYSIS

Now that we've examined the structure and purposes of the financial statements, we can use that information to inform us and help us in our analysis. Since most important decisions involve a concern for the financial impact of the outcome, we should give this aspect of analysis some degree of emphasis. Be sure to gather all of the relevant and current financial statements (including the notes to the financial statements) and any other related information to begin a systematic analysis of the financial health and status of the organization. Again, this is often done in determination of the fiscal feasibility of a venture to either remedy a problem or pursue an opportunity on behalf of the organization.

PRELIMINARY ASSESSMENT AND PREPARATION

Much can be learned simply by looking at financial statements. Now that we've gained an understanding of what the various elements of the statements mean and what value they have, we can get a general impression of financial status and performance just by comparing some numbers.

For example, if we were interested to know what the solvency of the organization is at a given point in time, we can look at the balance sheet and examine the current assets. We can also view the cash flow statement to look at cash receipts, cash from operations, and ending cash balance. These, coupled with the gross profit from the income statement, give us a pretty good idea how the organization is doing relative to solvency.

On the other hand, if we were to look at the current liabilities on the balance sheet, the operating expenses on the income statement, and the cash disbursements (and possibly the net borrowings) on the cash flow statement, we could appreciate the current expenses that the organization is facing.

Even looking at the bottom line of each of the statements will help us in formulating a general picture of the financial status of the organization. If the total assets and total liabilities on the balance sheet, the net income amount on the income statement, and the ending cash balance on the cash flow statement all reveal an excess of assets, income, and cash on hand, expending money to solve a serious problem is much less of an immediate concern.

However, although helpful, these general assessments may not be as fully informative as we may need. For that reason, we should consider some specific financial assessment techniques. Often of great value are the financial ratios.

FINANCIAL RATIOS

Financial ratios are mathematical comparisons of various elements of the financial statements that help to reveal relationships and possible influences of those elements. They are generally categorized as ratios of liquidity, resource management, profitability, or **leverage**. Financial ratios are not absolute and are not stand-alone assessments. They should always be considered jointly and in concert with other financial and operational information. Remember: Any insights gained from financial ratios are relative. The list of financial ratios is almost endless, but for the purposes of organizational or system analysis within EMS, we will explore only the most prevalent and useful ratios here.

Liquidity Ratios

Liquidity ratios are often the most popular of the financial ratios because they provide immediate feedback as to the solvency of the organization (often an important concern to any analyst). Liquidity ratios tell the analyst how readily convertible assets are to cash.

Current Ratio. One of the more popular liquidity ratios is the current ratio. This ratio compares the current assets to the current liabilities in an effort to show the financial strength of the organization and the safety of the debt holder's claims at present. It is derived solely from the balance sheet and calculated as follows:

$$\text{Current ratio} = \frac{\text{Current Assets}}{\text{Current Liabilities}}$$

The ratio generally hovers around 2:1, whereas a higher ratio (above 2:1) represents better solvency and a safer organization that has a financial cushion. If the current ratio is 2:1 or better, there is considerable safety. But, as the ratio nears a 1:1 relationship, the organization is barely able to meet its current financial obligations. Keep in mind, too, that high **current ratios** may also indicate poor management practices, particularly in lost investment opportunities and idle cash reserves.

Quick Ratio or Acid Test. Another common liquidity ratio is the **quick ratio**, also known as the acid test. By comparison to the current ratio, the quick ratio is a more stringent assessment as it examines *components* of the current assets that are even more liquid. It is also derived solely from the balance sheet and is calculated as follows:

$$\text{Quick Ratio} = \frac{\text{Cash} + \text{Marketable Securities} + \text{Receivables}}{\text{Current Liabilities}}$$

This ratio is closer to a 1:1 relationship since you are examining only the most liquid of assets in comparison to what is often a much larger current liabilities. Most often, the ratio is a fraction of 1:1 relationship, such as a 0.80:1 ratio. The closer the ratio is to a 1:1 relationship or greater (e.g., 1.5:1), the more likely the organization can meet financial demands immediately. In fact, the quick ratio is a good tool for determining how well an organization can respond to a major crisis during which immediate cash is critical.

Resource Management Ratios

Resource management ratios deal with assessing the effectiveness of the management and utilization of the organization's assets. For service-oriented industries, like EMS, resource management is less of a factor than for production companies that rely on sales of products. Nonetheless, we'll explore a few aspects of resource management.

Asset Turnover Ratio. This assessment is typically applied to sales in a production company, but it can be modified to have some application to a service industry like EMS. In lieu of sales, the ratio can examine the level of services in relation to the amount of asset turnover for the organization. In determining the **asset turnover ratio**, we are examining the efficiency of asset utilization based on a level of service delivered. By comparing the gross revenues from services rendered to the amount of gross assets, we can get a rough estimate of asset utilization. From the income statement we can derive the net or gross revenues from services, and from the balance sheet we can obtain the gross assets. The formula would look like this:

$$\text{Asset Turnover Ratio} = \frac{\text{Gross Revenue from Services}}{\text{Gross Assets}}$$

Ratios of less than 1:1 suggest a small amount of assets are needed to generate revenues, whereby ratios greater than 1:1 indicate that a large asset reserve is likely necessary to support the level of services produced. Large ratios may also suggest that asset depreciation could be great and equipment upgrading might be in order.

Accounts Receivable Outstanding. A somewhat atypical measure of resource management, this assessment is not quite a ratio, but it is included here as a form of resource management analysis. Again, this is an adaptation of the concept in sales, modified to have applicability to services. The assessment attempts to measure the *age* of the outstanding accounts receivable. If accounts that are yet to be paid are found to be very old, there is a strain on resources that are necessary to support the delivery of services. Accounts receivable that have a short turnaround time free up assets and allow maximal utilization of resources. Thus, this becomes a measure of resource utilization.

This measure is derived by obtaining the accounts receivable from the asset side of the balance sheet and multiplying that dollar amount by the days in the year that service is provided (for most EMS organizations, that number is 365), then dividing that product by the annual net services from the income statement. In formula format it appears as this:

$$\text{Receivable Outstanding Days} = \frac{\text{Receivables} \times 365 \text{ (Days)}}{\text{Net Services (Annual)}}$$

This will yield the average number of days the organization's accounts receivable is outstanding. Shorter days outstanding reflect a good collection rate for the organization.

Profitability Ratios

Profitability ratios help to determine an organization's **return on assets** or services delivered, which is a measure of the agency's ability to earn a profit, which is different from liquidity. Liquidity measures are important indicators of an organization's short-term financial health and ability to respond to a crisis. Profitability reflects that organization's long-term health and ability to survive. It is entirely possible for an organization to be profitable without having immediate reserves to fend off a crisis. In general, profitability ratios compare the organization's net profits with another financial parameter.

Since most EMS organizations are not publicly traded, we will forego the return on equity ratio (a popular ratio in publicly traded organizations) and focus, instead, on the return on assets, the **return on services** (commonly referred to return on sales), the gross margin ratio, and the profit margin ratio.

Return on Assets. Here we'll examine how well the organization utilizes its assets to generate revenue. A simple (but important) ratio, we need only to obtain the net income from the bottom of the income statement and divide it by the total assets from the balance sheet to arrive at the return on assets (ROA). The formula should look like this:

$$\text{Return on Assets} = \frac{\text{Net Income}}{\text{Total Assets}}$$

The return on assets is the easiest form of profitability analysis and is usually depicted as a percentage (multiply the result by 100 and add the percentage symbol). The higher the percentage of ROA, the better are the indications that the assets are yielding income. An agency with a low ROA may not be running as efficiently as it should.

Return on Services (Sales). **Return on services** is typically applied to the sales of a production company, but we'll modify it here to help reveal profitability in the EMS service industry. This is another useful analytical tool for determining profitability by examining what percentage of revenue from services results in net income—otherwise known as a **profit margin**. It, too, is of a simple construction. The net income from the bottom of the income statement is divided by the net services from the top of the income statement. The result tells how much income is yielded from the revenue generated by services. The formula is simple:

$$\text{Return on Services (Profit Margin)} = \frac{\text{Net Income}}{\text{Net Services}}$$

This measure is also often reported as a percentage (multiply result by 100 and add percent symbol). Combined with the ROA, these measures reveal a great deal about an organization's profitability. A high return on services (ROS) suggests a high profitability from services delivered—certainly a goal of most organizations.

Gross Margin. Gross margin is slightly different than return on assets or return on services as a measure of profitability. It reveals how much of the revenue from services is realized as profit, or conversely, what does it cost for operations? Consider that if the net services (revenue generated from services delivered in the review period) is measured against the gross profit (both from the income statement), it would reveal how much profit is made from the services delivered. To look at it from the opposite perspective, the difference between the net services and the gross profit is merely the cost associated with the delivery of those services. Thus, it also reveals how much an organization profits after the cost of operations is removed—a measure of what it costs to make money.

In formula format, gross margin should appear thus:

$$\text{Gross Margin} = \frac{\text{Gross Profit}}{\text{Net Services}}$$

This measure is a simple, but valuable, relationship between revenue and profit. It is also reported as a percentage. High percentages of a gross margin indicate very little cost goes into generating revenue for the organization. This, too, could be considered a measure of operational efficiency (with some limitations, of course).

Leverage Ratios

These ratios pertain to financial leverage, or the effort of an organization to maximize financial outcomes—whether results in gains (intentional) or losses (undesirable). The manner in which most organizations accomplish this is through loans and investments. An organization can leverage its equity by borrowing against it or utilizing some of its assets to acquire fixed assets (sometimes associated with risk). One important consideration of leverage is the amount of debt burden an organization has to its lenders. Although there are many **leverage ratios** (many that deal with equity and stock), we'll focus on those that have the greatest applicability to most EMS organizations.

Debt Ratio. Perhaps the most useful of the leverage ratios for EMS organizations, the **debt ratio** reveals how much debt an organization has against its total assets. Clearly, a high debt ratio is a very risky situation, for it means that the organization's assets may barely cover the debt burden the organization has at the time.

To determine the debt ratio, obtain the current and long-term debt amounts from the balance sheet and combine that amount. Then divide that sum by the total assets of the organization (again, from the balance sheet). This will indicate the amount of assets necessary to cover the total debt. The formula is simple:

$$\text{Debt Ratio} = \frac{\text{Total Debt (Current + Long-term Debt)}}{\text{Total Assets}}$$

This result may be written either as a number (decimal) or as a percentage (multiplied by 100). The higher the percentage, the greater the amount of assets necessary to cover the debt. This is the kind of information important to a lender and, therefore, important to you as an analyst trying to determine if the organization can handle more debt to resolve a problem or capitalize on an opportunity. It is important to recognize that this analysis does not take into account depreciation of assets or liquidation values of assets—so, it is an approximation of debt ratio.

Interest Coverage. **Interest coverage** is a very useful measure to determine the relationship between the net profit of an organization and its interest payment amounts. The value of this measure is that it helps one to understand the ability of the organization to meet its current debt load. Revenues will fluctuate, but debt interest generally remains the same. So, when revenues are down, the interest coverage may reveal some level of risk.

To best assess interest coverage, it is important to use the net earnings (net profit) or the income from operations on the income statement. This is the earnings (net services), less the cost of services and the incidental, marketing, and general expenses, as well as any income interest or taxes. When we consider income or earnings before interest and taxes, we are taking a most conservative approach. This amount is referred to as earnings before interest and taxes (**EBIT**) and is a commonly applied concept in financial matters. For the sake of our discussion, EBIT can be the income from operations from the income statement. If so, the formula should look like this:

$$\text{Interest Coverage} = \frac{\text{Income from Operations}}{\text{Interest Paid}}$$

Note: The denominator for this measure is the amount of interest paid, not the interest rate.

This measure is often recorded as a number, not a percentage. That number represents the number of times the income from operations can cover its debt service obligations. For example, if the income from operations was $12,000 for the month of July and the amount of interest paid on the loans amounted to $120, the interest coverage would be 100 times.

Financial ratios can be a very useful tool in the financial analysis of an organization. They must always be considered in the context of other information, particularly all of the financial statement including footnotes, the apparent overall health of the organization, the type of organization and the kind of business it does, and the mission of the organization. Some organizations may normally operate on the edge of revenue loss or debt burden, but most should have a solid financial foundation from which to operate. To help put the financial statements and financial ratios into perspective, several other analyses should sometimes be considered.

BREAKEVEN ANALYSIS

Breakeven analysis is an economic analytical process whereby an organization's business activity is determined at the juncture of profit versus losses—in other words, "At what point does the organization make money or lose money on its operations?" We will once again modify this principle, typically applied to sales production, to help us in our analysis of the EMS service industry. Breakeven analysis is a form of **operating leverage**, whereby altering operational practices can create financial advantages.

To effectively apply this principle and understand this concept, we must first understand **fixed costs** versus **variable costs**. Fixed costs are those costs in an organization that do not change with the level of service provided. For example, if you were paying a mortgage on a building to house your operations, a call volume increase of ten, twenty, or a hundred calls in a day would not increase the mortgage costs. Fixed costs often include payments on a loan, interest on a loan, depreciation of capital goods, salaries of support staff (to a limited extent), marketing costs, and the acquisition of capital goods (also to a limited extent). It is important to recognize that fixed costs do not need to be fixed over a lifetime, nor can they not fluctuate. Many fixed costs increase or decrease over time, but the key aspect is that they should *not* be tied directly to service volume.

Variable costs, on the other hand, *are* tied to volume. They are the costs associated with delivering additional services. A good example in the EMS industry would be fuel costs. If you delivery ten, twenty, or a hundred more calls in a day, then your fuel costs for the ambulances will go up. Other variable costs may include soft supplies, oxygen utilization, medication stock, crew salaries (to an extent), and other operational supplies. Again, the key is that variable costs are tied to an increase in operational volume.

Thus, volume appears to be the key aspect to cost determination for breakeven analysis. This is very true. In fact, we have just identified the major components of breakeven analysis as they relate to volume: They are price, fixed costs, and variable costs. Of these, fixed costs have the least to do with volume changes, but they must be considered in breakeven analysis.

Let's begin our exploration of breakeven analysis by examining fixed costs. We know that fixed costs can fluctuate somewhat and can even disappear (or increase) over time. We can consider fixed costs without taking these variations into consideration with no ill effects. So, let's say that your EMS organization has accrued about $15,000 in fixed cost each month, between loans, interest payments, clerical support staff, and other non-operational costs. If we were to graph that amount over time, it would look like the graph in Figure 4.7.

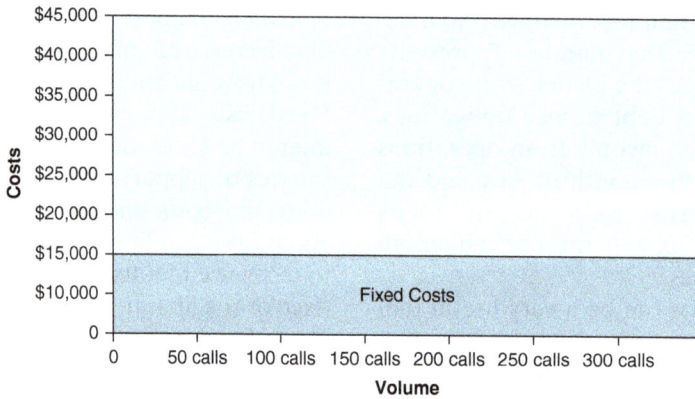

FIGURE 4.7 ■ Fixed costs in WeCare EMS.

The costs would essentially remain the same throughout the review period. Now, let's add to that the variable costs. To do so, we must consider volume since variable costs go up in conjunction with an increase in call volume. For illustrative purposes, let's say that variable costs go up proportionally with increases in call volume (we know this isn't true as an increase in ten calls in a day does not demand an increase in salaries, for example). For simplicity, let's say that variable costs go up $3,000 for each 100 volume of calls increase. The graphic depiction of the variable costs, as described, is illustrated in Figure 4.8.

As you can see, the variable costs are added to the existing fixed costs and are directly related to increases in the volume of calls. From this, one can surmise that an increase in call volume is associated with a known increase in **total costs** (Total Costs = Fixed Costs + Variable Costs). Thus, we have accounted for everything except for the price component. Let's now examine that aspect.

Price is commonly assigned to the sale price of a product. Since EMS does not sell products, but rather delivery services, let's replace *price* with *fee*. This parameter can be associated with the average fee that a customer

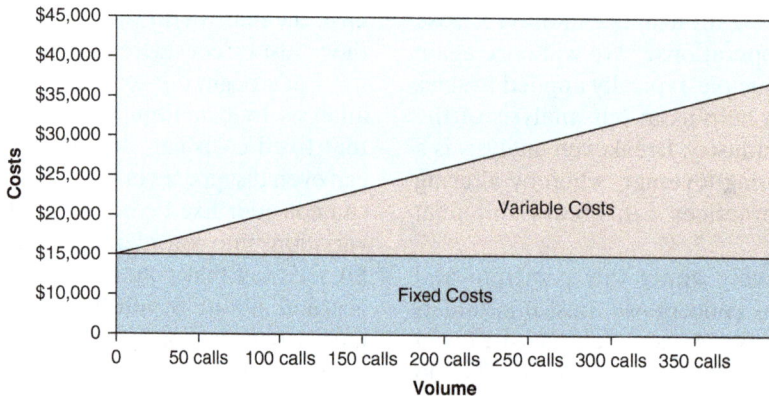

FIGURE 4.8 ■ Variable costs in WeCare EMS.

must pay for the delivery of EMS services. Again, we'll try to keep this simple for illustrative purposes, so we'll consider an EMS service fee that is average for basic life support calls and advanced life support calls regardless of transportation distances or supplies utilized.

WeCare EMS has always tried to keep prices low for its customers and charges only $150 per call on average. Based on this fee structure, the service has managed to turn a small profit, but it cannot expand. At what point does the organization make a profit based on call volume, and what kind of call volume would be necessary to generate enough revenue for expansion? These questions can be answered by plotting the average fee per call on the variable and fixed costs graphs. This line is represented in red in Figure 4.9.

From this illustration, we can see that a small call volume is necessary to cover total costs (about 140 calls). After that, much of the operations revenue contributes toward more profit (as long as the fixed costs remain the same and the variable costs increase at the established rate). The point at which revenue exactly covers all expenses is termed the **breakeven point**: Above this is profit, below it are losses. This relationship of volume, cost,

and fee structure can be represented by the following formula, where "I" represents the profit the organization earns, "V" is the volume of calls, "P" is the fee charged for each call, "VC" is the variable costs, and "F" is the fixed costs:

$$I = VP - (VC + F)$$

Simply put, if you deduct the total costs (variable cost plus fixed costs or VC + F) from the product of the fee charge per call and the total volume of calls (VP), your profit is revealed.

Similarly, the breakeven point (in volume of calls) can be expressed as a formula. This is represented when "I" (profit) is at zero. In this formula, "C" represents the unit variable cost—that is, what the variable cost is to deliver one EMS call. It would be written:

$$\frac{F}{P - C} = V$$

To increase profit, one would consider increasing volume, but remember that also increases cost (sometimes at the expense of profit). You can also increase profit by reducing costs (a practice performed by many organizations). Often, you will find that the greatest profit can be realized when fixed

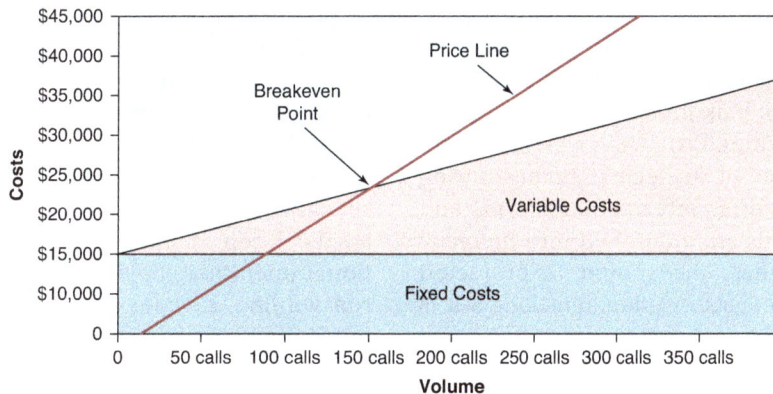

FIGURE 4.9 ▨ Price line and breakeven point for WeCare EMS.

costs are reduced rather than reducing variable costs or increasing volume.

There is a lot more to breakeven analysis, but this simple introduction may help you to consider how call volume can influence profit when costs (variable and fixed) are known. Breakeven analysis can assist you in determining the feasibility of an organization to incur additional expenses and, in particular, whether or not to consider increasing fees to cover new ventures or expansions. The one aspect that breakeven analysis does not answer is the impact that raising fees has on volume. This is another economic principle that is important, but outside the scope of this chapter. Interested readers are encouraged to explore additional information on breakeven analysis in the References section at the end of this chapter.

OTHER FINANCIAL ANALYTICAL CONSIDERATIONS

Examining the financial statements and using that information, both in raw form and in financial ratios, can be very revealing and helpful in decision making. However, at least two other considerations deserve mentioning with regard to the financial aspect of your analytical approach. They are **pro forma statements** and **time value of money**.

Pro Forma Statements
Pro forma statements are traditional financial statements that look forward or project future financial activities. Pro forma statements are often a product of strategic planning, during which short-term, intermediate-term, and long-term goals are quantified into financial expression. These are similar to projected operational budgets, but should include assets and other traditional components of financial statements.

Pro forma financial statements typically include a pro forma balance sheet, a pro forma income statement, and a pro forma cash flow statement. They are informed speculations on projected financial performances of the organization.

Pro Forma Balance Sheet. The pro forma balance sheet projects future assets and liabilities. There is often a considerable amount of freedom in these projections, but they should be based on reliable speculation. If the strategic long-term plan is for expansion of services to include neighboring communities and the anticipated increase in call volume is 80 percent, then a projected pro forma balance sheet can be generated based on existing knowledge of financial performance. Whatever modifications are made to the pro forma balance sheet, they must correlate to the pro forma income statement in the exact same manner. Increased earnings and costs on the pro forma income statement should be demonstrated equally as assets and liabilities on the pro forma balance sheet.

Pro Forma Income Statement. Owing to the nature of projection and speculation of operational activities, the pro forma income statement is usually prepared first. As one derives the strategic goals and translates them into financial performances, the revenue and costs of operations can be reasonably projected. This simulation will result in an approximation of a future (pro forma) income statement. From that, other financial projections can occur. It is much easier to estimate projected revenues (and operating costs) from increased run volume than it is to estimate increases in assets. Keep in mind that projecting additional operating activities not only increases run volume, revenues, and operating costs, but it may also have associated increases in general and administrative costs and the need for additional financial leverage in the form of loans and interest.

Pro Forma Cash Flow Statement. Pro forma cash flow statements are largely a product of the pro forma income statement and the pro forma balance sheet. When the ending balances of two or more pro forma balance sheets of different periods demonstrate a marked difference, we can illustrate that difference in pro forma income statements and pro forma cash flow statements. The pro forma cash flow statement will reveal the cash flow that will result from the projections.

The process of developing pro forma statements is not much different from the traditional financial statements, other than the well-grounded speculations. The same assumptions and rules should be followed throughout their development. Pro forma statements can be extremely helpful in estimating costs and revenues for any future problem resolution or opportunity for growth.

Time Value of Money

A familiar phrase is "A dollar doesn't buy what it used to." This is a statement that has its basis in reality. The value of money *does* change over time as the value of goods and services change. This concept is considered the **time value of money** and is the basis of determining net present values. It is fairly easy to see the difference in the time value of money when we consider the cost of a single item 20 years ago compared to today, but does a year or two make a difference as well? Well, it depends on how much money and in what manner it is being considered. Valuing money over time to determine **present value** and future value is a fairly complex and sometimes lengthy process. We will explore the fundamentals here in this chapter and leave expanded understanding of these concepts to the prerogative of the reader.

Depending on circumstances, money can appreciate, depreciate, or be considered equivalent to other valuable goods. To illustrate appreciation of money, we'll be using a simple example of time value of money by examining compounding interest. We know that compounding interest is the appreciation of the value of money over time at a specified rate of interest. For our example, we'll use a 5 percent interest rate that is compounded annually only (not a typical situation, but it illustrates the concept well).

Let's say we have $100 and want to invest it. If we put it in the bank to earn that 5 percent interest, in 1 year we'll have $100 plus 5 percent interest or,

$$\$100 \times (1 + 0.05) = \$105$$

The money appreciated over time (1 year) to $105. Now, let's consider this same situation if the individual chose *not* to invest that money but, rather, decided to hold onto it for 1 year. Obviously, in 1 year he would have $100. In this instance, we could ask "How much money would he need to have right now to invest so that in 1 year he would have that same $100?" This question underlies the concept of present value. For it asks "What is the present value of $100 1 year from now?" The means of determining that present value is similar to our compounding interest example. Instead, we will determine the value of the $100 by reversing the interest (sort of). We'll take the $100 and determine what amount of money at an interest rate of 5 percent would be necessary to start with 1 year prior? We can do that by the following formula:

$$\text{Present Value} = \frac{\$100}{(1 + 0.05)} = \$95.24$$

We can confirm this by asking "How much money would I have in 1 year at a 5 percent annual interest rate if I invested $95.24?" To determine that, simply use our compounding formula:

$$\$95.24 \times (1 + 0.05) = \$100 \text{ (or very close)}$$

What determining present value enables us to do is to value present money for the future. If we know we need $10,000 in 2 years, how much do we need now to invest at a given interest rate? The easiest way to make that calculation is to simply add an exponent to the parenthetical expression in the denominator that is equivalent to the number of years. To illustrate, using the above example:

$$\text{Present Value} = \frac{\$10,000}{(1 + 0.05)^2} = \$9,070.30$$

This concept of determining the present value of future money is termed **discounting future value**. We have discounted the $10,000 into the equivalent present value (of $9,070.30).

Let us now consider the opposite effects of the time value of money. What happens when something of value loses value over time or depreciates? Probably the best examples in EMS are ambulances and capital equipment. If we purchase an ambulance today, we will list it on our balance sheets under assets, but what will its value be 10 years from now? To determine its future value, we need to depreciate it.

Several methods can be used to depreciate physical goods, but each must be acceptable to current accounting standards and prevailing IRS rules. Let's begin with the most common and least complex method: **straight-line depreciation**.

Straight-line depreciation is simply a process of taking the current value of the item (what was paid for it) and estimating its useful life, and its value at the end of its useful life (if we were to resell it). If a piece of equipment costs us $12,000, it has a useful life of 6 years, and the value of the equipment is about $2,000 at the end of 6 years, we can use the straight-line depreciation method to estimate its annual value for each year.

This is done by taking its present value (cost) and deducting its end-of-life value and dividing that amount by the years of expected life. In our example,

$$\$12,000 - \$2,000 = \$10,000 \text{ then,}$$
$$\$10,000/6 \text{ years} = \$1,666.66$$

For each year, following the first year, we will then deduct the $1,666.66 amount. So, at the end of the first year, it will be valued at $10,333.34 ($12,000 − $1,666.66). The next year, $1,666.66 will be deducted from that amount, and so on. Figure 4.10 illustrates the depreciation for the life of the equipment.

Another concept of depreciation is **accelerated depreciation**. This approach is useful for assets that depreciate at a nonstandard rate, such as ambulances. An ambulance,

---

Cost of Equipment: $12,000
Expected Life of Equipment: 6 years   End-of-Life Value: $2,000

Year	Depreciation	Value	Accumulated Depreciation
1	$1,666.66	$10,333.34	$1,666.66
2	$1,666.66	$8,666.68	$3,333.32
3	$1,666.66	$7,000.02	$4,999.98
4	$1,666.66	$5,333.36	$6,666.64
5	$1,666.66	$3,666.70	$8,333.30
6	$1,666.66	$2,000.04	$9,999.96
Total:	$9,999.96		

FIGURE 4.10 ■ Straight-line depreciation example.

much like a car, will depreciate more quickly in the first few years than its later years of life. For this reason, depreciation should occur at a more rapid rate in the beginning years. There are commonly two forms of accelerated depreciation: **double-declining balance depreciation** and **sum-of-years depreciation**.

In double-declining balance depreciation, the straight-line depreciation rate is doubled for the life of the item beginning with the first-year balance and continuing for every year balance thereafter. For example, using our $12,000 piece of equipment as before, we know that the rate of depreciation is ⅙ per year or 16.7 percent. We double that amount in the first year to 33.3 percent and depreciate the cost value of the equipment by that amount ($3,996) as follows:

$$\$12,000 \times 33.3\% = \$3,996$$
$$\$12,000 - \$3,996 = \$8,004 \text{ depreciated value}$$

From here, we depreciate each end-of-year balance by the same rate of depreciation (33.3 percent). Figure 4.11 illustrates the depreciation using the double-declining balance method.

From Figure 4.11, you can see the rapid depreciation of the value in the first years. But, as the useful life of the equipment nears the end, the depreciation amount is much less.

The remaining accelerated depreciation method to consider is the sum-of-years depreciation approach. Here the focus is on the years of useful life the equipment has. That number is sequentially added to itself from beginning to end to arrive at a sum of sequential years. For example, if the useful life of a piece of equipment were 6 years, we would sequentially add those years together as follows:

$$1 + 2 + 3 + 4 + 5 + 6 = 21$$

That number now becomes the denominator in the annual depreciation rate for the equipment, with the numerator being the actual year number in reverse order. These concepts applied together would result in the following annual depreciation rates:

$$6/21, 5/21, 4/21, 3/21, 2/21, \text{ and } 1/21$$

So, the order for those rates of depreciation would be:

Year 1: 6/21 or 28.57 percent

Year 2: 5/21 or 23.81 percent

Year 3: 4/21 or 19.05 percent

Year 4: 3/21 or 14.29 percent

Year 5: 2/21 or 9.52 percent

Year 6: 1/21 or 4.76 percent

Cost of Equipment: $12,000 End-of-Life Value: $2,000
Expected Life of Equipment: 6 years Rate of Depreciation: 33.3%

Year	Depreciation	Value	Accumulated Depreciation
1	$3,996.00	$8,004.00	$3,996.00
2	$2,665.33	$5,338.67	$6,661.33
3	$1,777.78	$3,560.89	$8,439.11
4	$1,185.78	$2,375.11	$9,624.89
5	$790.91	$1,584.20	$10,415.80
6	$527.54	$1,056.66	$10,943.34

FIGURE 4.11 Double-declining balance depreciation example.

Cost of Equipment: $12,000

End-of-Life Value: $2,000

Expected Life of Equipment: 6 years

Rate of Depreciation: varies by year

Year	Rate	Depreciation	Value (less end-of-life value)	Accumulated Depreciation
1	28.57%	$2,857.00	$7,143.00	$2,857.00
2	23.81%	$2,381.00	$4,762.00	$5,238.00
3	19.05%	$1,905.00	$2,857.00	$7,143.00
4	14.29%	$1,429.00	$1,428.00	$8,572.00
5	9.52%	$952.00	$476.00	$9,524.00
6	4.76%	$476.00	$0	$10,000.00

FIGURE 4.12 ■ Sum-of-years depreciation example.

This approach will also depreciate the equipment in an accelerated depreciation fashion with the greatest depreciation in the beginning years. The result is illustrated in Figure 4.12 for comparison to the other methods.

Figure 4.12 depicts the present value (cost) of the equipment at $12,000 and the end-of-life value at $2,000. The amount to be depreciated is the difference, or $10,000. Using the sum-of-years depreciation method, the $10,000 remaining value is depreciated by the rate in the table depending on the year and the accumulated depreciation is summed. So, for example, in the fourth year, the value of the equipment is $1,428.00 and the amount depreciated is $8,572.00, which would total $10,000 (the current depreciated value plus the amount depreciated).

Additional methods of depreciation and certainly many more concepts are related to the time value of money. Some, like the net present value (NPV), is fairly complex but important for financial analysis. Readers are encouraged to investigate NPV through the references listed at the end of this chapter.

EMS-Specific Analysis

Several financial analysis approaches have specific benefit to EMS delivery of services. Most are adaptations of production or service indicators of performance and may have value in assessing EMS efficiency.

One very popular assessment is the **unit hour utilization analysis (UHUA)**. This has been proposed as an effective means of measuring productivity and helping to determine overall operational costs for delivery of services. However, this measure has come under considerable scrutiny, particularly if it is not sufficiently inclusive of costs and utilization (Fitch & Associates, 2005). To understand this performance measure, let's look at the components. The unit hour is the time interval of 60 minutes in which the ambulance is fully equipped and ready for service—it is fully operational. By comparison, the utilization measure is the time in which the ambulance is being fully utilized—delivering services. Utilization will be a component of unit hour since the ambulance must be available, fully equipped, and staffed in order to be utilized. Therefore, utilization will be a percentage of the unit hour. If utilization occurs in 35 minutes of every hour the ambulance is available for service, the unit hour utilization rate is 58.3 percent.

Clearly, most EMS agencies will endeavor to maximize their unit hour utilization rate. Having a utilization rate of 50 percent or more would indicate high efficiency of assets. This would suggest high productivity and effective utilization of resources. To affirm this prediction, simply take your cost of services from the cash flow statement and apply that to the call volume for the specified period of time under analysis. This operational cost could then be compared to the results of your breakeven analysis, gross margin ratio, return on services ratio, and the unit hour utilization analysis times the cost of services product.

Variances of this measure may also prove to be useful. Once costs of services are derived from the cash flow statement, it can be used to compare unit hour costs (cost of services/unit hour), costs per transport (cost of services/

total transports in period), or other cost assessments. Similarly, the net income amount from the cash flow statement can be used to determine revenue per transport by simply dividing the net income value by the number of transports in the period.

Many other permutations of utilization analysis can be applied to EMS in the delivery of services. When assessing utilization, be sure to keep in mind the hidden costs, incidental costs, and opportunity costs when using this to make decisions. Each assessment should be thoroughly thought out before declaring an outcome.

Best Practices

Financial Analysis in an EMS Course

With the advent of a greater scope of practice and professional accountability in health care overall, there is an inherent need for improved financial performance of EMS organizations. This advancement is new to the EMS professions, and formal preparation is essential for future successes. One institution of higher education that is providing instruction to EMS leaders and managers is Central Washington University (CWU). Along with

other courses in clinical development and EMS leadership, Financial Analysis in EMS is offered through an online, distance education format. The EMS Paramedicine Program at CWU offers an Advanced Standing option for practicing paramedics to achieve a Bachelor of Science degree in Paramedicine that enables effective leadership in the profession.

For more information, please visit the Central Washington University (CWU) website.

CHAPTER REVIEW

Summary

In the course of analysis for EMS system problems or entrepreneurial ventures, the most commonly emphasized analytical approach is that of financial analysis. Although properly designed analyses should have their foundation in research methodology, often the most sought-after component is the financial analysis. Therefore, almost all analytical

approaches have some element of financial analysis. Determining feasibility is often a matter of cost. Exploring opportunities is often a matter of profit or reward. Conducting a well-designed financial analysis, based on the examination of financial statements, interpreting relationships among the financial statements, conducting analysis through financial ratios, examining or developing pro forma statements, conducting breakeven analysis, and applying the time value of money concepts will often yield the most informative analytical results. This, coupled with the research findings and perhaps cost-benefit analysis, impact analysis, or feasibility analysis, will provide the most effective solution and a high confidence level for decision making.

WHAT WOULD YOU DO? Reflection

The situation that you face may not be as daunting as you may think. You've requested the financial statements from your organization's financial accountant and examined the balance sheet, income statement, and statement of cash flows for several periods. From this, you see that the trend that is developing with increased growth has also been revealed in your growth of retained earnings. Your debt burden is actually quite small and your fixed assets have grown over the years. You conduct several liquidity ratios, and they all show a sizable amount of money that is available for a down payment on the new ambulance. You also conduct a debt-to-assets ratio, determine your interest coverage, and find your organization is in good standing for increased debt.

The pro forma statements that you've requested show a continued trend toward organizational growth and the opportunity for asset investment now with little future risk. Your breakeven point is far below your current fee for services. You feel confident that making this purchase and financing the expense is a good financial decision and will provide for future growth.

Review Questions

1. If you were interested in learning how much cash money your organization could assimilate in short order, how would you determine that?

2. In your financial analysis of your organization, you discover that there is a fairly substantive amount of outstanding collections yet to be paid by customers. How would you regard that portion of outstanding payment, and where would you expect to find it on the financial statements?

3. A competing EMS organization in a nearby community is soliciting services at one of the local hospitals and several long-term-care facilities. To fend off this operational threat, you decide to develop and dispense marketing materials. The print/copy vendor has recently billed you for those services. Where would you expect those costs to appear in your financial statements?

4. In financial terms, how does net worth differ from working capital?

5. What areas of financial decision making does the cash flow statement reveal with regard to the traditional business model?

6. With regard to the operational component of the cash flow statement, on what three areas does this section focus?

7. How can the financial statements and their constituent parts be tied to organizational improvement and strategic planning?

8. Compare and contrast the features and characteristics of the three financial statements.

9. Which of the liquidity ratios is the most stringent and why?

10. The financial analysis of your organization revealed that the current ratio is 3.8:1, the asset turnover ratio is 0.8:1, and the return on

assets performance is 34 percent. However, the return on services is almost 90 percent. What might be surmised from these findings?

11. You learn that your competing EMS agency has a receivable outstanding of 65 days, whereas yours is just less than 43 days. Which organization is doing better?

12. During routine financial analysis of your organization, you discover that your interest coverage rate is only 1.6. What does this mean to you, and what action should you take, if any?

13. You decide to conduct a breakeven analysis of your organization. In your analysis, you discover that your fixed costs are about

$68,000 per month and your variable costs are an additional $44,000 per month on average. Your call volume has a minimum of six calls per day, a maximum of fifteen calls per day, and a mean of nine calls per day. Your average fee for service is $443 per call. How good is your price structure?

14. If the current interest rate is 1.51 percent for a 5-year certificate of deposit with a minimum deposit of $10,000, how much money would you earn at maturity if the interest were compounded annually?

15. How much money would you need to invest today to earn $100,000 in 3 years at 3 percent interest?

References

Fitch & Associates, LLC. (2005, Fall). "Does UhU Accurately Measure Workload?" *Management Focus: for Providers of Emergency Medical Services 20*(3), 1–2.

Helfert, E. A. (2003). *Financial Analysis Tools and Techniques: A Guide for Managers.* New York: McGraw-Hill.

Ittelson, T. R. (2009). *Financial Statements, Revised and Expanded Edition.* Pompton Plains, NJ: Career Press.

Mayes, T. R. (2012). *Financial Analysis with Microsoft Excel,* 6th ed. Independence, KY: South-Western CENGAGE Learning.

Key Terms

accelerated depreciation A method of asset depreciation that places larger portions of depreciation in the early years of the expected life of the item either for accounting or tax deduction purposes.

accounts payable Appears on the balance sheet and represents obligations the organization has to creditors and suppliers.

accrued expenses Expenses that have come to term or have been already incurred; a sum of all the current expenses.

accumulated depreciation Appears on the balance sheet as the total depreciation of all assets for the period under review.

asset turnover ratio A financial ratio that demonstrates the effectiveness at which assets in the organization can generate service revenue.

assets On the balance sheet, assets are tangible items that have associated value; often of property, buildings, and equipment.

balance sheet One of the more commonly utilized financial statements; it reveals the values of the assets, liabilities, and shareholder's equity at a given point in time.

breakeven analysis An analytical process that determines at what point the revenue of services covers all of the costs of operations (fixed and variable costs).

breakeven point In breakeven analysis, the exact point where revenue or retained earnings meet the total costs of operation; where there is no profit and no losses.

capital stock The investment into a business for start-up and add-on growth by owners of the company.

cash disbursements Found on the cash flow statement, payments made to vendors that lower the cash asset and the accounts payable sections of the balance sheet.

cash flow statement A financial statement that tracks the movement of cash through an organization over a period of time; focuses on operations, investments, and financing.

cash receipts Also referred to as collections, the item on the cash flow statement that reveals the cash received from doing business.

costs of services Typically costs of goods sold on the income statement in production companies; those costs and expenses associated with the production or delivery of services.

current assets Found on the balance sheet, the items of value that are expected to be turned into cash in the short term (usually less than 1 year).

current debt On the balance sheet under the liabilities column, the portion of debt that is due for collection in the short term (usually under 1 year).

current liabilities Found on the balance sheet, current liabilities are bills that are due in the short term (usually under 1 year) and typically consist of accounts payable, accrued expenses, current debt, and income taxes that are currently due for payment.

current ratios A common measure of an organization's liquidity that relates the sum of the current assets to the sum of the current liabilities.

debt ratio Also known as the debt-to-assets ratio, reveals an organization's outstanding debt obligations to total assets; used as a measure of financial leverage.

discounting future value A means of applying the concept of time value of money whereby the present value of future money is determined.

double-declining balance depreciation A method of depreciation of goods whereby the depreciation rate of the good is doubled for the expected life of the asset; a means that places the greater depreciation in earlier years for an accelerated depreciation.

EBIT Earnings Before Interest and Taxes; a measure of money revenue that is conservative.

ending cash balance Found on the cash flow statement, it represents the final registration on the statement; the result of the beginning cash balance, plus any cash received, and minus any cash spent.

equity Found on the balance sheet, the recorded ownership claim of common and preferred stock for an organization's stakeholders.

fixed asset purchases Found on the cash flow statement, the amount of money spent purchasing assets (property, buildings, and equipment).

fixed assets Found on the balance sheet, properties or items of value to the organization that are not intended for sale and usually used over and over again in the production of services (or sales).

fixed costs Any cost that doesn't vary in value or amount with changes in operations over time.

GAAP Generally Accepted Accounting Procedures; procedures, conventions, and practices that are established by the Financial Accounting Standards Board (FASB) for the preparation and reporting of financial statements.

general and administrative expenses Found on the income statement, costs not directly associated with the delivery of services or operations; often a significant source of indirect expenses; includes administrative expenses, clerical, preparation, and day-to-day costs such as utilities.

gross margin Found on the income statement, it represents the amount of money left over from the revenue of services delivered minus the cost to deliver those services; also called gross profit.

gross profit Found on the income statement, it represents the amount of money left over from the revenue of services delivered minus the cost to deliver those services; also called gross margin.

incidental services Sometimes found on the income statement, representing services provided that are not directly linked to the mission of the organization, but may have value and even generate income.

income from operations The revenue generated by the activities purposed by the organization in its delivery of services; derived from the gross margin minus the operating expenses.

income statement One of the financial statements that provide information on the revenues and matching costs for an organization during a specific time period; a report of the income earned by the organization; sometimes referred to as an operating statement or profit and loss statement.

income taxes payable Part of the current liabilities on the balance sheet that indicates the current tax liabilities.

interest coverage A financial analysis tool that reveals the relationship of periodic interest expense to operating income before or after taxes; often used to judge an organization's ability to pay interest on loans.

interest on income Earnings outside of operational income, often from interest on investments or cash dividends.

leverage The practice of using organizational resources (usually assets or equity) to achieve greater profits or revenue; a means of magnifying the profits from increases in the volume of services through fixed assets or equity; usually either operating leverage or financial leverage.

leverage ratios Financial analysis tools that measure how much of the company's assets are financed with debt to demonstrate an organization's "equity cushion" and how much the organization can tolerate additional debt.

liabilities A category on the balance sheet that illustrates the obligations the organization has to its creditors and vendors.

liquidity The ability to convert assets (current) to cash in the short term; also known as solvency.

liquidity ratios Financial analytical tools that demonstrate an organization's ability to convert current assets to cash in the short term.

long-term debt Any financial payment obligation that extends beyond 1 year.

long-term liabilities Expenses to an organization that extend beyond 1 year in duration; often found on the balance sheet.

net borrowings Found on the cash flow statement, it is the difference between any new borrowings in a time period and the amount already paid back.

net current assets The current assets of an organization less the current liabilities; also known as working capital.

net income The final registration on the income statement that reveals either a positive cash reserve or a negative cash loss; the difference between the combined income from operations (gross margin less operating expense) and interest income and the amount paid out in taxes.

net sales (or net services) Found on the income statement, the amount of revenue earned in a period of time from sales (in a production company) or services delivered (in a service company).

net worth The recorded value of shareholder's equity on the balance sheet; same as shareholder's equity.

non-cash transactions Financial exchange activities that do not involve cash flow; activities that may involve action, but do not immediately add to the cash on hand and will not appear on the cash flow statement.

operating expenses Found on the income statement, those expenditures that a company incurs in its operations to earn income; often includes service delivery, marketing, incidental services, and general and administrative expenses.

operating leverage The effect that changes in volume of services from operations has on profits caused by fixed costs; any change in operational practices that offers financial advantages.

present value The value today of a future asset or sum of money calculated by discounting the future value to today's value.

pro forma statements Financial statements that project revenues and costs based on formulated conditions and trended expectations over a period of time.

profit margin A financial performance measure derived by comparing the net services from the income statement with the net income; sometimes referred to as gross margin.

profitability ratios Financial analysis tools that relate profits to some other component of financial information; often referred to as "return on" ratios as they reveal the profit return on another financial aspect.

quick ratio A financial analysis tool (also known as an acid test) that is very effective in revealing an organization's liquidity.

retained earnings The accumulated amount of past and current earnings of an organization that are not disbursed (either maintained as a cash asset or invested into the organization).

return on assets A financial analytical tool that reveals the relationship of an organization's earnings to its total assets as a measure of productivity or profitability; abbreviated ROA.

return on services A financial analytical tool for determining profitability by examining what percentage of revenue from services results in net income; known as return on sales in a production organization.

revenues The money earned by an organization through the delivery of services and other sources of income; an elemental aspect of the income statement.

shareholder's equity Found on the balance sheet, the recorded value of residual claims of all of the owners of the organization.

straight-line depreciation A method of depreciation that is traditional and progressively depreciates the asset or good over the useful lifetime of the asset, less the recovery or end-of-life value; the depreciation is equivalent for each year depreciated.

sum-of-years depreciation A method of depreciation that places greater emphasis on the depreciation of an asset or good in the earlier years of its useful lifetime by fractioning the depreciation in accordance with the number of useful years as a depreciation rate.

time value of money A financial concept that recognizes that money changes value over time (typically a reduction toward the future) and enables financial and economic analysts to value future amounts of money in present-day equivalencies.

total assets Found on the balance sheet, all of the assets of an organization, including the current assets, fixed assets less depreciation, and all other assets owned.

total costs An economic principle used in breakeven analysis that includes all variable and fixed costs of an organization.

unit hour utilization analysis (UHUA) A performance measure adapted from the manufacturing industry for application to EMS that assesses efficiency of utilization of services per unit of time.

variable costs The costs in an organization that are associated with operation and are subject to fluctuation in amounts coincident with the changes in volume of services.

working capital The amount of earned income that an organization has generated that is available for expenses, investments, and new acquisitions; derived by deducting current liabilities from current assets; also known as net current assets.

Cost-Benefit Analysis

5 CHAPTER

Objectives

After reading this chapter, the student should be able to:

5.1 Demonstrate an understanding of the purpose, applicability, and components of cost-benefit analysis.

5.2 Describe the basic elements of cost-benefit analysis with regard to monetization, benefits, costs, and net benefits.

5.3 Describe the differences between cost-benefit analysis and cost-effective analysis and how each applies to the analytical approach.

5.4 Describe each of the basic steps to a cost-benefit analysis, how each is applied, and how each influences subsequent steps.

5.5 Demonstrate an understanding of impacts, how to quantify impacts, how to monetize impacts, and how to determine their present value and future value in the time value of money.

5.6 Describe the social discount rate and how that relates to net present value and the cost-benefit analytical approach.

5.7 Demonstrate an understanding of the sensitivity analysis process, including Monte Carlo sensitivity analysis, how that can be applied, and what relevance that has to the cost-benefit analysis process.

5.8 Demonstrate an understanding of the theoretical premises of valuing a human life, what options exists, what a statistical life is, how it applies to welfare economics, and how to apply these concepts to cost-benefit analysis.

5.9 Describe the meanings of Pareto efficiency and the Kaldor-Hicks criterion and how they can be applied to cost-benefit analysis.

Key Terms

cost-effectiveness
   analysis
ex ante cost-benefit
   analysis
ex post cost-benefit
   analysis
future value
impact analysis

impacts
in media res cost-
   benefit analysis
inputs
Kaldor-Hicks criterion
monetization
Monte Carlo
   sensitivity analysis

net benefits
net present value (NPV)
outputs
Pareto efficiency
present value (PV)
public good
quality-adjusted life-
   years (QALY)

regulatory impact
   analysis
sensitivity analysis
social discount rate
statistical life
time value of money
welfare economics

WHAT WOULD YOU DO?

You are trying to decide how to best spend a recent windfall of $25,000 that was donated to your organization for equipment. You are trying to choose between a new monitor-defibrillator, some new capnograph devices, a fiber-optic laryngoscope, and a portable ultrasound device. The opinions of the crews vary considerably, and there seems to be no consensus. Choosing to rely on analysis, you have held focus group interviews. The focus interviews produced a recurrent question that continues to nag you: "Which of these devices will save the most lives?" Even if you could determine that answer, how would you value it? What would be the best approach?

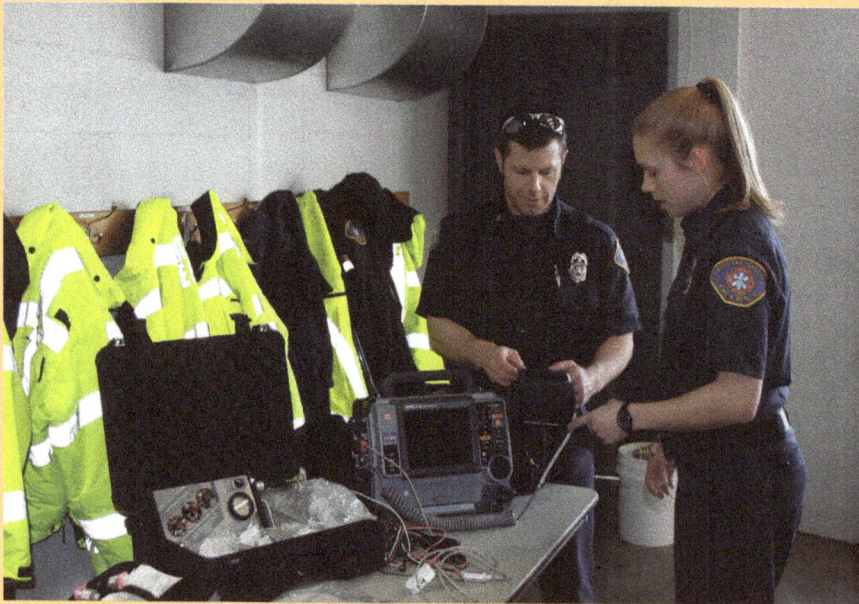

FIGURE 5.1 ■ Making a choice.

INTRODUCTION

With every analytical approach to a problem or opportunity, the initial process begins with proper problem identification, followed by establishing a firm foundation of the analytical process based on established research principles. Most often, that analytical template is followed by a financial analysis.

Financial analysis is essential to most problems or projects as the matter of cost is often foremost in an organization's list of concerns. However, simple accounting costs based on financial statements may not be enough — there is often a need to consider other costs that are either not present on the financial statements or difficult to value.

Prime examples might include **impacts** of a project, problem resolution, or opportunity for growth. If the impact has yet to occur, it will not appear on the financial statements. Sometimes, these impacts are positive; sometimes they are negative. In either case, they can affect the decision as to whether or not to proceed with the resolution, opportunity, or project. Other examples can include the impact these initiatives may have on the organization, the community, or society in general. When considering the purchase of an expensive piece of equipment, such as a monitor-defibrillator, we often justify the expense by claiming it will save many lives. So, how do we quantifiably measure that consequence? Many of these situations cannot be fully realized until they are well underway — in which case, they may result in regret in retrospect. How can we anticipate their influences? How can we approximate the societal benefit they produce? How can we better assist our decision making with this nebulous information? It may be time to turn to cost-benefit analysis.

Cost-benefit analysis (CBA) is a process of valuing or monetizing impacts of an event, initiative, policy implementation, problem resolution, or similar venture and determining their net benefit — that is, comparing the initiative's benefits to its costs. Some prefer to place the emphasis on the benefits of such analysis and term the process benefit-cost analysis, but it remains the same process. Here, we will refer to it by its common nomenclature of cost-benefit analysis.

An impact is any consequence from the initiation or implementation of a project, solution, or venture. In order to be treated as an impact in CBA, there must be a cause-and-effect relationship between an outcome of the project, solution, or venture and any individual(s). Impacts can be many and of a very diverse nature. Impacts may have a positive consequence to the project or initiative (benefit) or a negative consequence (cost). If a piece of equipment improves patient care by reducing morbidity or if a new process or procedure improves an organization's revenues, they are considered benefits. If a new medical device creates an additional demand for supplies or specialized training or if an organization's expansion into a neighboring community necessitates greater staffing, they are considered costs. A single project or initiative may even have both costs and benefits associated with each impact.

THE BASICS OF COST-BENEFIT ANALYSIS

The general process behind cost-benefit analysis is cataloging the impacts of a project or event into comparable benefits or costs. This is often all encompassing and considers any conceivable impact, both positive and negative. Those impacts are then valued (designated some form of quantifiable value), most often through **monetization**. Monetization is a process of placing a money value on the impact. Once monetized, the impacts can then

Best Practices

Cost-Benefit Analysis Becoming a Standard

A careful search of the literature reveals that more and more EMS systems and city administrators are employing a cost-benefit analysis to justify added tax levies, expansion of services, and opportunities for mergers.

This necessity is likely resulting from greater municipal accountability to the public and elected officials. Knowing how to effectively and accurately conduct a CBA is critical, not only to solicit additional funds but also to ensure efficient operations.

Some examples of CBAs conducted in EMS include the following:

- *Olympia Washington for delivery of services. (See the Olympia Washington website.)*
- *NHTSA, EMS Technology Assessment Template. (See the organization website.)*
- *Sterling Heights Fire Department in Michigan for delivery of services. (See the organization website.)*

These, and other similar studies, illustrate the utility and structure of typical CBAs for EMS.

---

be summed, collectively on the positive side and on the negative side, and the results compared to one another. This process is termed **net benefits**. Desirably, the benefits will outweigh the costs. If they do, the project or resolution may proceed forward; if not, it may be abandoned.

The information gained from cost-benefit analysis (when properly conducted) is extremely valuable. It may tip the scales in a decision whereby, financially, the costs may be higher than desired, but the true benefit from the venture will justify its expense. The opposite may also occur. The financial analysis may reveal the costs are reasonable, but the cost-benefit analysis fails to demonstrate a true benefit in the venture. Therefore, cost-benefit analysis will often follow the foundational analytical inquiry and the financial analysis of the problem or initiative.

Cost-benefit analysis has garnered so much appreciation that any federal project or regulatory provision with a monetary impact of $100 million or more requires a cost-benefit analysis (Whitehouse.gov, 1993). The U.S. federal government first mandated the general use of CBAs in Executive Order 12291, issued by President Ronald Reagan in early 1981 (Boardman, Greenberg, Vining, and Weimer, 2001). Virtually all federal agencies now conduct CBAs on a regular basis to demonstrate feasibility of the adoption of most policies and regulatory guidelines. In government parlance, CBAs are often referred to as **regulatory impact analysis** since they typically involve the impacts of regulatory policies.

IMPORTANT DISTINCTIONS REGARDING COST-BENEFIT ANALYSIS

Often, one will be interested in whether or not a venture, policy, or project will be effective based on its associated costs. Basically, "Will this venture be worth the expense?" In this process, we often evaluate the benefits monetarily through the outcomes and compare those monetary values with the costs of executing the process, but we fail to consider the societal benefits. Or, we can measure the impacts of an initiative, but cannot monetize all of them realistically (as is often the case with health care, where saving a life or reducing morbidity is difficult to value in terms of money). In these circumstances, we are constrained from conducting a true cost-benefit analysis, as a CBA necessitates that we measure and monetize all benefits. We are, therefore, measuring only the effectiveness of the initiative and not all of the benefits. We term this approach, a **cost-effectiveness analysis**. This is an important distinction. In cost-benefit analysis, we *must* be able to measure *all* impacts and monetize them to determine the net benefits.

So, in cost-effectiveness analysis, we measure the associated costs of a venture, but compare them to a nonmonetized effectiveness measure instead of societal benefits. Most evaluations we do to determine whether or not a venture is worth the costs are likely cost-effectiveness analyses.

Cost-effectiveness analysis may be very valuable, but often is of less value than cost-benefit analysis. The reason for this is the lack of monetization of the benefits. As mentioned previously, many initiatives, major equipment purchases, or new interventional practices in health care often present with this type of challenge. For example, if we were to consider purchasing a portable ultrasound device for our EMS agency, would the expense justify the cost? It could be argued that employing such a device may facilitate field diagnoses and reduce morbidity and save lives—a reasonable argument. However, how can we monetize that outcome? This is a difficult matter that we will address later in this chapter, but it is alternatively reasonable to simply declare an estimated "saved lives" could be

realized by utilization of a portable ultrasound device. In doing so, we can compare the cost of the equipment to the number of saved lives to determine its cost-effectiveness, but that would not be placing a monetary value on human life.

Although cost-effectiveness analyses and similar approaches have value, we will focus our attention on cost-benefit analysis in this chapter as it often provides greater value toward decision making. For this reason, we will need to monetize all costs and benefits in our analysis in order to make fair comparisons.

TYPES OF COST-BENEFIT ANALYSES

We can categorize cost-benefit analysis into three types. The first to consider is the most common and usually the most applicable type: *ex ante* **cost-benefit analysis**. In this type, we are attempting to determine the costs versus benefits of a project, solution, or initiative *before* the project, solution, or initiative is begun. This approach is particularly useful in determining whether or not to proceed with a venture before costs are incurred.

The second form of cost-benefit analysis is the *ex post* **cost-benefit analysis**. Here, we would conduct cost-benefit analysis *after* the event, initiative, or solution has already been concluded. Since it is not preemptive, it contributes little toward decision making, but it does provide affirmation that the project was beneficial.

The third type is termed *in media res* **cost benefit analysis**. This form of cost-benefit analysis is conducted *during* the implementation of the project, initiative, or problem resolution. This type has characteristics of both *ex ante* and *ex post* cost-benefit analyses. In some instances, two or more forms of CBAs are conducted as comparisons (e.g., conducting an *ex ante* cost benefit analysis and an *ex post* cost-benefit analysis to compare outcomes).

Since the process is essentially the same for all three types, we will focus on the *ex ante* cost-benefit analysis form in this chapter. Components of the process can be modified to accommodate the other types as needed.

■ THE BASIC STEPS OF CONDUCTING A CBA

Conducting a truly effective cost-benefit analysis requires a systematic, methodical approach that may appear daunting at an initial glance. But, if we break the process down, we can execute the entire process into isolated and interrelated steps. The most popular and highly regarded authority on cost-benefit analysis suggests that this process consists of nine steps (Boardman, Greenberg, Vining, and Weimer, 2001). Each of those steps is described here in a sequential, progressive manner.

STEP 1: SPECIFYING THE ALTERNATIVES

Each time we consider conducting a cost-benefit analysis, we should be contemplating several alternative solutions or approaches. Whether it is seeking solutions to a problem, examining varying ways to develop an opportunity for growth, or looking for different ways to launch an initiative, considering alternatives is the foundational approach to cost-benefit analysis. Figure 5.2 illustrates a simple example of the benefits and costs associated with expansion of services into a neighboring community.

As illustrated in Figure 5.2, the organization is contemplating expansion into the neighboring community through three alternatives. The first is to purchase outright the building necessary to house the crew and ambulance in the coverage area of the neighboring community. The second option is to rent an existing building for temporary housing of the crew and equipment. The third alternative is to facilitate an outsourcing of services from an existing, for-profit EMS agency under contract. Each of these three alternatives is listed in Figure 5.2. Now, we can proceed to the next step of deciding which of the possible benefits and costs should be considered in our analysis.

STEP 2: DECIDING WHICH BENEFITS AND COST COUNT

Following the listing of alternatives, we now begin listing benefits and costs that can potentially be realized in this venture. The list may be lengthy, but it should be pared down to the most relevant. In Figure 5.2, only the most relevant benefits and costs are listed.

In this scenario, the reduction in response times considers only the operating benefits of crew availability for more rapid turnaround times, subsequent increased call volume, and a reduction in missed calls. In this simple example, there is no consideration for the societal benefit for the improved response on the general health and well-being of the community. In addition, some intangible benefits are not monetized, such as increased goodwill in the community, improved morale among the crewmembers, and future opportunities that this venture could engender.

Additional benefits in Figure 5.2 include the projected increased call volume from the expansion, the newly acquired fixed asset of the purchased building, the additional revenue from municipal retainer fees from the

	Purchase new building	Rent existing building	Shared service with other EMS
Benefits			
Operational cost savings from a reduction in response times	$12,000 (based on estimates of known information)	$12,000 (based on estimates of known information)	$6,000 (based on estimates of known information)
Increased call volume (est. at 4,500/year)	$1,350,000	$1,350,000	$675,000
Retained fixed asset	$450,000	None	None
Annual municipal retainer fees	$30,000	$30,000	$15,000
Savings from reduced travel time	$5,600	$5,600	$3,000
Total Benefits	**$1,847,600**	**$1,397,600**	**$699,000**
Costs			
Purchase of building	$450,000	None	None
Interest on loan	$20,250	None	None
Additional crews	$278,640	$278,640	$139,320
Reallocation of EMS unit (ambulance)	$8,110	$8,110	$8,110
Increased marketing demand	$450	$450	$450
Operational expense	$15,550	$15,550	$10,110
Administrative & general expenses	$18,120	$18,120	$12,045
Total Costs	**$791,120**	**$320,870**	**$170,035**
Net Benefits	**$1,056,480**	**$1,076,730**	**$528,965**

FIGURE 5.2   Sample cost-benefit alternatives list.

newly established contract, and the savings from a reduction in travel costs due to the additional station. There may be more benefits to consider, but we'll use only these for illustrative purposes.

The associated costs include the cost of the new building purchase, the interest on the mortgage loan, the cost necessary to staff additional crews, the cost to reallocate existing resources (ambulances and equipment) to the new site, and the financial costs of an additional marketing demand for the adjoining community. Again, some other costs may be considered, but we'll limit our concerns to those listed.

STEP 3: CATALOGING THE IMPACTS AND CHOOSING MEASUREMENT INDICATORS

By listing the impacts as either benefits or costs, we have cataloged those impacts. There is one other aspect that deserves some clarification. Impacts may be either **inputs** or **outputs**. An input would be any asset or factor that contributes to the development of the venture, whereas an output would be any product or result of that venture. An example of an input might be the cost of the building or increased revenue from an increase in call volume. An example of an output might be the savings in travel expenses or the reduction in missed calls.

Now that they are properly cataloged, we can begin choosing how we intend to measure the impacts. The cost savings from a reduction in response times can be determined through the positive change in call volume subsequent to the expansion (if conducted *ex ante,* this measure would need to be projected), the inclusion of otherwise missed calls, and the reduction of overtime where it might be affected by delayed call response.

The item of additional calls generated by the new coverage area is fairly straightforward, but it would need to be projected if the CBA is *ex ante*. The value of the purchased building and the amount of the contract retainer fees are also straightforward in their measurement. The savings from a reduction in miles traveled would require some computation of estimated reduction in response distances, but that can be fairly well approximated.

The cost of purchasing the building, the interest on the loan, the estimated additional cost to employ additional crews to staff the new station, the additional cost to supply and relocate one of the existing ambulances (the purchase of a new ambulance to meet this new demand would replace this item on the impact list), and the increased costs to provide marketing to the new coverage area can all be reasonably well measured.

STEP 4: PREDICTING THE IMPACTS QUANTITATIVELY

This step may require some degree of insight and vision (some would say imagination, but we *do* try to ground our claims with factual information). Here, we need to approximate (if the CBA were conducted *ex ante* as it likely would) the values of the impacts. For example, the additional crews necessary to staff the ambulance in its new station could be calculated from known information, such as the number of EMTs and paramedics necessary to staff the unit and the number of hours each crew member would be scheduled. The same approach can be made for some of the other impacts, such as estimating the increase in call volume based on known population density of the new coverage area and the associated call rate. The same information can inform the increased demand for marketing as well.

In many CBAs that involve changes in human outcome, whether it is a change in utility, health, or survival, this step may be the most challenging. It is often difficult to predict how many lives the new monitor-defibrillator will save or how much better the crews will be able to field-diagnose patients using a portable ultrasound device. It may now be somewhat obvious that cost-benefit analysis is not always a precise process. Some of the necessary information may need to be extrapolated or approximated from known, foundational information. This is representative of some of the acknowledged shortcomings of this process, but it is important nonetheless.

STEP 5: MONETIZING THE IMPACTS

In this step, we take the values that we've determined from our measurements of the impacts and place a monetary value on each of them. Some impacts are measured in monetary terms, like the purchase of the building or the increase in marketing demand or staffing. Others are measured in other quantitative units and must be valued monetarily (monetized) to be considered in cost-benefit analysis. In the end, all impacts must be monetized.

If, for example, we were to determine that the expansion of services into the neighboring community would improve response times and deliver improved EMS services that would result in better outcomes for the citizens, we would then need to value quantitatively that outcome. Let's say that this expansion is predicted to save three lives per year (such an estimate should not be arbitrary, but based on a grounded theory that can be found in many health policy or health economics textbooks or other sources). We would then be required to monetize that outcome. What value does three lives have? That matter is addressed in the *Valuing Human Life* section of this chapter.

For our example, we would monetize the operational savings, the revenue from the increased call volume, the value of the building, the retainer fees, and so on. Each cell of the cost-benefits alternative list table should contain a dollar amount, if applicable. These values are entered into our table in Figure 5.2. As noted, not all impacts apply to each alternative. For example, if the alternative chosen is to rent a building, there is no fixed asset to monetize.

STEP 6: DISCOUNTING THE BENEFITS AND COSTS TO DETERMINE PRESENT VALUE

Simply placing a monetary value on each impact is not enough. Since these cost-benefit analysis endeavors typically occur over time, we may need to discount the future-day values to present-day values. This necessity is a product of the natural process of monetary values diminishing over time—a concept commonly referred to as **time value of money**. Items of value in the future tend to cost more than they do in the present because of this reduction in the value of money. If we could purchase an item in the future with today's money, it would cost us less than future money. Let's say you wanted to buy a $100 stethoscope (**present value [PV]**) 5 years from now. In that future year, that price might be $110. If it's the same

quality of stethoscope, you could have purchased it for $10 less today. Now, imagine the opposite scenario. What if we wanted to buy a stethoscope that we somehow know will cost $110 in 5 years? We would need to have only $100 today to buy it. What this represents is two different perspectives of the same purchase. The difference is the value of money at two different times. This concept is often difficult to conceptualize, so give it some thought and imagine variations of it. This principle is the same in reverse—that is, how much money would we need today to earn $110 5 years from now if the average interest rate was 2 percent? The answer is $99.63.

In cost-benefit analysis, we need to know **future value** in present-day terms. So, future benefits and costs are discounted to present-day values. This step would not apply if the CBA were conducted with no regard to the life of the project, solution, or venture.

The process of discounting future values can be somewhat complex, and readers interested in the multiple aspects of this concept are encouraged to explore the "References" section at the end of this chapter. For our purposes now, we'll examine the basic discounting principles.

In some instances, a benefit or cost may not be realized until sometime in the future. To determine what value that benefit or cost has in present-day terms, we can calculate it by knowing what year we are interested in and knowing what the **social discount rate** currently is. Knowing the current social discount rate presents somewhat of a challenge. It is a fiercely debated issue among analysts and often a bit contentious. Some of that debate stems from the fact that the social discount rate will vary year to year, and the life of most projects, solutions, or ventures spans at least several years. Even in government, the current social discount rate may vary among agencies and departments. Most folks, these days, seek the current social discount rate via the Internet. Some suggestions are also offered in the "References" section at the end of this chapter. Most social discount rates hover around 7 percent which, realistically, might be a bit high (Boardman, Greenberg, Vining, and Weimer, 2001; Friedman, 2002; Wikipedia.org, 2013). There is a fairly wide range of social discount rates among countries, with poorly developed countries having higher social discount rates (since costs tend to escalate at a faster rate in developing countries).

Once the social discount rate is determined, calculating the present value (PV) is quite simple. If the future cost or benefit value is known, the present value is determined by dividing it by the social discount rate raised to the power of the year it exists:

$$PV = \frac{Cost}{(1 + r)^{year}} \quad or \quad PV = \frac{Benefit}{(1 + r)^{year}}$$

where r is the social discount rate and the year is the exponent.

Let's apply this to a real-life example. If a piece of equipment will cost $2,000 5 years from now, and we know the social discount rate is 6.5 percent, then we calculate the present value as follows:

$$PV = \frac{Cost}{(1 + r)^{year}} \quad or \quad PV = \frac{\$2,000}{(1 + 0.065)^5}$$

The PV (cost) is then equal to $1,459.76 at that social discount rate (6.5 percent) for 5 years in the future.

Determining the future value (FV) of a present-day cost or benefit is simply the reverse. Instead of dividing the cost (or benefit) by the social discount rate raised to the power of the year, we multiply it:

$$FV = Cost(1 + r)^{year}$$

or

$$FV = Benefit(1 + r)^{year}$$

So, if the cost of a piece of equipment is $12,000 today, knowing the social discount

rate (technically, in this case it's known as the compound interest factor) is 6.5 percent, we can calculate the future value 3 years from now as follows:

$$FV = Cost(1 + r)^{year}$$

or

$$FV = \$12,000(1 + 0.065)^3$$

The future value will then be $14,495.40 at that compound interest rate (6.5 percent) for 3 years in the future.

For multiple-year calculations, this discounting procedure simply follows a series of the same basic equation. The result of each equation is summed to produce the total.

In cost-benefit analysis, we need to determine the **net present value (NPV)**—the difference between the total sum of benefits minus the total sum of costs. If we were to determine the NPV of the combined benefits and costs in the current year, we would simply add all of the benefits (represented in this example as B) and all of the costs (or C) and find the difference ($B - C$). That difference is the NPV. The challenge lies in estimating the NPV of future years. For that, we need to include a discount rate. That rate can be represented by r and indicates the discount rate for that particular year. So, if we wanted to know the NPV of the benefits and costs *next* year, we could estimate it by the following equation:

$$NPV = \frac{B - C}{(1 + r)}$$

Now, to discount beyond the next year, we simply raise the denominator to the power of the year in the future. For example, if we wanted to know the NPV of the benefits and costs 3 years from now, the equation would look like this:

$$NPV = \frac{B - C}{(1 + r)^3}$$

Let's use some numbers to illustrate the result. The total benefits of a proposed project have been monetized and total $145,000. The total costs are $120,000. Therefore, the net benefits are $25,000 (benefits minus the costs). Based on a discount rate of 7 percent, the NPV of that amount 3 years from now is this:

$$NPV = \frac{\$145,000 - \$120,000}{(1 + .07)^3}$$

$$NPV = \frac{\$25,000}{(1.07)^3}$$

$$NPV = \$20,407.45$$

That means that the future value of the present-day net benefits is $20,407.45. This represents the present-day amount of money discounted by the social discount rate for 3 years from now. Put another way, if we wanted the net benefits to be valued at $25,000 3 years from now, we would need to have $20,407.45. This reversal of perspective represents the difference between discounting of money to compounding of money.

This process leads us to the next step in cost-benefit analysis, which is really nothing more than a logical conclusion of our efforts thus far.

STEP 7: COMPUTING THE NET PRESENT VALUE OF EACH ALTERNATIVE

This step is somewhat simple. Now that we know the monetary value of each of the impacts and have discounted them over the life of the project, solution, or venture, we can now sum that amount to determine the NPV of each of the alternatives.

Again, this step would be unnecessary if the CBA were focused on a single year or event. This step only has utility when we want to approximate a discounted value over time. One might be hesitant to even apply these discounting principles in cost-benefit analysis, given their uncertainty and debatable nature. In fact, applying discount rates to future values is even varied and contentious among government agencies and not uniformly applied (Zerbe, Han, Layton, and Leshine, 2002). Nonetheless, its application to a CBA is strongly encouraged as it provides a much more meaningful value to outcomes and provides greater precision and reliability in decision making.

In application to our example in Figure 5.2, we simply take the total benefits and total costs for each alternative, calculate their net benefit, and determine their NPV based on the principles discussed previously. An example is illustrated in Figure 5.3.

	Purchase new building	Rent existing building	Shared service with other EMS
Benefits			
Total Benefits:	$1,847,600	$1,397,600	$699,000
Costs			
Total Costs:	$791,120	$320,870	$170,035
Net Benefits	$1,056,480	$1,076,730	$528,965
NPV @ 7% for 3 yrs.	$862,402.38	$878,932.41	$431,793.01
NPV @ 7% for 5 yrs.	$614,880.98	$767,693.61	$377,144.73

FIGURE 5.3   Determining net present values of each alternative.

STEP 8: PERFORMING A SENSITIVITY ANALYSIS

When we conduct a cost-benefit analysis in accordance with the steps described and the guidelines recommended, we accept some degree of estimation, projection, and uncertainty in our predictions. This may be obvious from our previous discussion regarding social discount rates, but it is especially true of CBAs conducted on health care–related purchases, projects, problem resolutions, or operational initiatives that involve patient care. It is generally very difficult to predict health care outcomes that result from any of these interventions. For this reason, we must conduct a **sensitivity analysis**. For the most part, a sensitivity analysis is a process of estimating our best guesses based on known histories and probabilities. A sensitivity analysis acknowledges the uncertainties by estimating the most likely outcomes based on probability statistics and making adjustments accordingly. The greater the degree of uncertainty in our predicted impacts, the more important sensitivity analysis is, and the greater is our risk of error in the final determination.

For many of you, this may sound familiar. Sensitivity analysis is very much akin to applying research principles to your analytical approach by using probability statistics to predict the most likely outcome. Similarly, it is also important in a process known as **impact analysis**. In some applications of research methodology to the analytical approach, we focus on a single variable by holding all other variables constant (or under control). The same approach can be adopted here. To determine how the net benefits might change over a period of time, we can vary a single assumption while holding all other assumptions constant (like the social discount rate). If all other assumptions remain unchanged and we alter the social discount rates for the intervention years of useful life of the project, we can then appreciate its individual impact. We are, in fact, conducting a sensitivity analysis of that single assumption. Probably the most common form of sensitivity analysis is termed a **Monte Carlo sensitivity analysis**. This will be the form that we will explore.

Let's begin by conducting a partial sensitivity analysis. What if we were projecting that the savings from a reduction in response times was $1,200 annually? Would that be sufficient for our purposes? Is that estimate accurate enough? How will the increase in call volume conversely affect the reduction in response times? To what extent will the reduction in travel times affect the reduction in response times? Each of these parameters can affect the savings amount from a reduction in response times. How do we account for those? There is where Monte Carlo sensitivity analysis comes in handy.

Monte Carlo sensitivity analysis provides a way of overcoming these uncertainties and unknowns. It is named thusly because it is similar to playing games of chance and using probabilities to predict likely outcomes. The process consists of three basic steps.

The first step is to identify each of the important uncertainties that have a quantitative value (typically impacts) and assign it a probability of distribution. For example, the average response time of our organization is 6.8 minutes currently. If our response distances from the new station are not much greater, our response times shouldn't vary too much from current estimates. We've projected an increase in call volume of approximately 4,500 calls per year with our expansion in the first year. In addition, we estimate that a reduction in travel times to adjacent regions of our coverage area to be about 2 miles for 20 percent of our current call volume. (Please keep in mind these are all estimated projections for illustrative purposes only.) This provides us with a start to our analysis. More complex methods are possible through statistical approaches, but we'll forgo them here.

The next step is to conduct a trial of the proposed estimates by randomly proposing a value from each of the parameters under consideration to compute the net benefits. To start, we should use the best estimated averages. In conducting this trial, we'll assume that all measures are evenly distributed (basically, that the mean and median are the same with equal distribution of possibilities to either side of the mean). Since these are the values originally logged in our cost-benefits alternative list table in Figure 5.2, this step is already completed. In future trials, we should derive randomly assigned values for each of the measured impacts that fall within a reasonable and expected range. This will be applied in the next and final step.

The final step is to repeat that same trial as many times as deemed necessary with varying values in the measured impacts using a randomly generated selection. The variances should be reasonable and expected, and the best results occur when only one input is varied at a time. We should avoid artificially inflating or deflating any values for the purposes of revealing a cause-and-effect phenomenon; we are interested in realistic projections, not influential variables. If we maintain a reasonably expected value range for each parameter, the law of averages will help us to determine which net benefit values will prove to be most likely.

The description and examples used here to illustrate sensitivity analysis are moderate in their complexity and difficulty. There are much more complex elements and methods that can be used to conduct sensitivity analysis and would demand a greater understanding of the process than described here. Comparatively, a sensitivity analysis may be as simple as varying one impact and estimating the consequence it has on the other impacts. Whichever approach you choose, be precise, modify the impact values based on grounded rationales, and minimize any biases or experimentations in the analysis.

STEP 9: MAKING A RECOMMENDATION

From each of the steps completed thus far, we can now offer a reasonable recommendation. Since most of the steps culminated in monetizing impacts, determining their net present value, and performing a sensitivity analysis, we merely need to base our recommendation on the determination of the NPV of the alternative and what preferences the sensitivity analysis indicated. Generally, the recommendation should be the alternative that had the greatest NPV, but remember that net present values are *expected values*. Although informative, they may not be exactly as predicted. Furthermore, the information provided by the sensitivity analysis might contradict the best choice, given the NPV. This inherent conflict is not uncommon and underscores the reason we must include *all* information regarding a choice or decision—so that we can choose the best alternative.

This recommendation is often made to principal authorities or leadership and, therefore, should be concise, convincing, and informative. It very well could be part of a larger proposal or recommendation that employs all elements of analysis. In doing so, be sure to systematically import all relevant elements in a fluent and logical manner that supports a final conclusion.

▓ VALUING HUMAN LIFE ─────

When conducting a cost-benefit analysis on health-related matters, we are often confronted with including the impact our alternatives have on human life. It may result in some improvement in living, a reduction of risk or disease, or even in saving lives. From an economic perspective, this necessitates valuing a human life—placing a dollar value on a human being. This is a matter of great debate and contention. Many would ask "How can you place a value on a human life? Life is priceless." As true as that statement is, we must look at it from other than a moral perspective.

Side Bar

CBA: Not as Simple as It Appears

The general, prescription for CBAs is to determine the net social benefits by deducting the costs from the benefits of a project or venture. Or, NSB = B − C where B = benefits and C = costs.

When this is applied to an individual, the results appear quite obvious. It is easy for one to examine all of the benefits that a decision might produce versus any costs that might be incurred. We use this premise in our everyday life.

It becomes more difficult when others are involved. And this is where CBAs are commonly applied. Consider this: Let's assume you were to examine a new practice or new venture that was likely to benefit most people involved. What about the impact it has on any others who might have a negative consequence?

From a pure, classical welfare economic perspective, the answer is easy: the benefits of many outweigh the losses of a few (a concept in utilitarianism from Jeremy Bentham known as "the greatest happiness principle"). But would you want to be the one that is disadvantaged? What voice do those unfortunate folks have?

The ethical dilemma this presents makes for difficult applications of CBAs sometimes. This can be further compounded by the difficulty of monetizing certain impacts (like loss or saving of life). So, it's not quite so easy sometimes.

ETHICS VERSUS WELFARE ECONOMICS

Normative ethics dictates that failing to promote or save lives is morally wrong. In fact, deontological ethics—a branch of normative ethics promoted by Immanuel Kant places emphasis on the act and intent of the person performing the act as the means of determining right from wrong and the "goodness" of the act. Based on these premises, the only right thing to do is to save one's life at virtually any cost. This ethical argument suggests that there can be no price placed on the human life. These types of ethical arguments form the basis of why EMS even exists: It is our moral obligation to help others. These are all very reasonable and sound arguments.

However, there are two additional perspectives that one should consider when contemplating the value of a human life in cost-benefit analysis. The first perspective is as follows: If the value of a human life is priceless, then by definition there can be no price placed on any given human life and, therefore, *all* expense should be directed at any effort to save a human life. I think we can all agree that this is unreasonable. How can a single human life demand all available resources? This means that given any sudden death situation, we should not stop resuscitative efforts regardless of the probable outcomes. This is not a standard practice in medicine. Medical practice is also directed by probabilities and pragmatic decision making. So, we can conclude that a human life (from a practical standpoint) is *not* priceless. This perspective needn't undermine our underlying beliefs—it simply provides a logical approach to practice.

The second perspective is more economic in nature. Economists who are well practiced with cost-benefit analysis are not interested in the true value of a human life—they are interested in the *statistical value* of a human life (otherwise known as a **statistical life**). In effect, this perspective attempts to determine how much an individual is willing to pay to reduce his risk of death. This is a measurable perspective and has everyday application. Any given person has a unique level of risk avoidance. There are folks who enjoy risky behavior (e.g., sky diving, deep sea fishing, and smoking). Even firefighting and law enforcement have inherent risks greater than that facing most individuals. Then, there are those who avoid risk at all costs Although this dichotomy seems straightforward, it can be a bit complex. For example, if given the choice to purchase a car with an airbag (e.g., an additional $500 per airbag), would you spend that much more money on a new car knowing that your risk is reduced during a crash? Many people might not opt to incur that additional expense. Fortunately, that matter is taken care of with federal regulations.

So, in conducting CBAs that involve human life, we might be best served by considering the statistical life of an individual. This is a principle that still generates some debate, but it is a well-accepted aspect of CBAs. It represents an important part of microeconomics known as **welfare economics**, whereby social welfare (an individual's well-being) is a central concept and concerns are on equality of distribution of goods and **Pareto efficiency** (discussed in the next section). There are various methods in applying these principles in cost-benefit analysis—some common to medicine as well.

One popular method of considering the value of human life is in **quality-adjusted life-years (QALYs)**. In cost-benefit analysis, this approach considers the effect some decision, intervention, or item acquisition has on the *quantity* and *quality* of one's life. From the quantity perspective, it determines how many additional years the event adds to the individual's life. From the quality perspective, it measures the change in the status of health the event provides to the individual's life. Both measures are complex and somewhat subjective. Interested readers are encouraged to explore additional information on QALYs in the "References" section at the end of this chapter.

Another approach is to statistically value a life over the entire lifetime based on productivity and contribution to society. This

approach may be the most unsettling and debated approach, but it does have some utility in welfare economics and CBAs. Depending on the source and the reason for determining the value of a human life, the monetary value of a human life varies considerably. Federal agencies are a common source of human life estimates with ranges from approximately $9.1 million as proposed by the Environmental Protection Agency for the impact that pollution has on human life (Associated Press, 2008) to $7 million by the Food and Drug Administration to $6 million by the Department of Transportation (Appelbaum, 2011). One Stanford University professor estimates the value of a human life to be approximately $129,000 per productive year of life (Kingsbury, 2008).

These estimates can be used in cost-benefit analysis for values of statistical life in determining monetary values for alternatives and sensitivity analyses. Currently, most authorities agree on a statistical life to be valued at around $7.9 million, with catastrophic causes (such as terrorism) a bit higher and death from chronic illnesses somewhat lower.

THEORETICAL FOUNDATIONS OF COST-BENEFIT ANALYSIS

As suggested earlier, cost-benefit analysis has its foundation in welfare economics, where the focus is on the well-being of individuals and an equal distribution of income and goods and services. A central tenet to welfare economics and cost-benefit analysis is the concept of Pareto efficiency.

PARETO EFFICIENCY AND THE KALDOR-HICKS CRITERION

The concept of Pareto efficiency is principled on defining efficiency such that any allocation of a good or service is considered to be Pareto efficient if no additional allocation alternative can make even one person better off without creating a disadvantage to another.

Some simple examples include the provision of a **public good**. A public good is anything that is nonrival in consumption; that is, one individual using it does not diminish it for another individual. Examples include the weather (enjoying the sunshine does not diminish it for others), or the ocean (at least for now), or goodwill. Public goods should also be nonexclusive—that is, available to everyone equally.

In terms of Pareto efficiencies, enjoying the sunlight, or enjoying the ocean, or experiencing goodwill from others does not diminish it for others and all can enjoy it without exclusion. Now, let's examine some practical applications of Pareto efficiency.

If one were to win the lottery, he would presumably become richer. Everyone can participate in the lottery, so it's nonexclusive. But, if you win, it diminishes the opportunity (and reward) to others to enjoy the same outcome, so it is *not* Pareto efficient. Winning the lottery disadvantages someone else (by them either not winning or winning a lesser amount).

In practice, very few policies, interventions, or public decisions are Pareto efficient. Virtually every decision will result in someone being either better off or worse off. For this reason, we strive to reach the "Pareto frontier" in hopes that most people will be better off than those who are worse off. This is the goal of cost-benefit analysis. If the net benefits of a project, problem resolution, or opportunity endeavor are positive, then it is considered to be Pareto improving (not quite efficient, but approaching it).

There is one other aspect of Pareto efficiency that deserves mentioning: the **Kaldor-Hicks criterion**. This involves a supplemental consideration to the concept of Pareto efficiency. We already know that an alternative should at least improve the lives of more

people than it makes worse off, but what if the margin is small? Is there any way to make improvement for those who will be made worse off? The Kaldor-Hicks criterion specifies that the alternative or endeavor can be chosen if those who will be able to benefit from the decision, resolution, or endeavor could compensate those who will be made worse off and still remain better off themselves after the compensation.

The Kaldor-Hicks criterion eases some of the restrictions of seeking Pareto efficiency in cost-benefit analysis. If one of the alternatives to a problem or opportunity can improve the lives of most people, and they, in turn, can somehow improve the lives of those less fortunate from the alternative, then it still remains a viable option. Let's consider a health care example for this concept.

Let's say you are in charge of the state health department and are interested in instituting an immunization policy that would benefit everyone who is immunized against the seasonal influenza virus strain. The problem is that some folks may object to (or not qualify for) the immunization for health, ethical, or religious reasons. Even though that may represent only a percentage of the state's population (say 20 percent), and most folks would benefit from the vaccine, there still remains that 20 percent who are vulnerable to the influenza virus. But your epidemiologist informs you that due to the concept of herd immunity, those who are protected from the virus will prevent the spread of the virus and the individuals who are not vaccinated will be at a much lower risk for acquiring the disease. In a manner of speaking, this represents the Kaldor-Hicks criterion and suggests that you should implement your immunization policy.

Although achieving Pareto efficiency is a lofty goal, it should nonetheless be our objective in any cost-benefit analysis that involves social welfare issues. Social welfare can even be translated into organizational welfare when the impacts are limited to the EMS organization or system. There are other aspects and concepts related to welfare economics to explore in the "References" section at the end of this chapter.

CHAPTER REVIEW

Summary

Cost-benefit analysis is often a critical component to any analytical approach that has an impact on others. Determining the best alternative solution to a problem or best option to consider for purchases or organizational growth are important matters and deserve the best possible outcome. Cost-benefit analysis enables an improved approach by examining the monetary values each impact has for each alternative and considering those impacts in comparison to one another with sensitivity analysis. In addition, understanding the future value of an impact (or, conversely, the present value of a future impact) may help in deciding between two or more alternatives.

In the end, we want what's best of all involved, so considering Pareto efficiency in our process of making choices and in decision making becomes quite important in the analytical process. It is equally important to recognize the true purpose of cost-benefit analysis, as well as its benefits and limitations, in deciding whether or not to employ CBAs and to what extent they should be employed. Once we've properly identified the problem, established the foundation of analysis through principles of research, conducted our financial analysis, and completed a cost-benefit analysis (if appropriate), we may then need to consider what impacts the choice or decision we've arrived at will have.

WHAT WOULD YOU DO? Reflection

The challenge that you're faced with is not an uncommon one. It is further complicated by determining which device saves the most lives and how the value of a human life figures into the decision. To remedy this challenge, you investigate the lifesaving potential of each device and research the current value of a statistical life. From this, you can list the alternative device choices to consider, list the benefits and costs of each, determine the net benefits, identify the impacts of each, monetize them (including the value of a human statistical life), perform a sensitivity analysis, and make a recommendation. In this instance, the pivotal issue is the number of human lives that could be saved with each device, which is then compared to the future value of the device, making the decision quite easy.

Review Questions

1. Why is a cost-benefit analysis important?
2. How does one derive net benefits?
3. How does cost-benefit analysis differ from cost-effective analysis?
4. How do *ex ante* cost-benefit analysis, *ex post* benefit analysis, and *in media res* cost-benefit analyses differ from one another?

5. Why is it necessary to monetize impact measures in cost-benefit analysis?
6. What does the time value of money represent?
7. How is net present value determined?
8. What is a sensitivity analysis, and how is it conducted?
9. How does the economic value of a human life differ from the social or ethical view of human life?
10. What is a statistical life?
11. What is Pareto efficiency?
12. What is the Kaldor-Hicks criterion?

References

Associated Press. (2008, July 10). "How to Value Life? EPA Devalues its Estimate." (See the MSNBC website.)

Appelbaum, B. (2011, February 16). "As U.S. Agencies Put More Value on a Life, Businesses Fret." (See the New York Times website.)

Boardman, A. E., D. H. Greenberg, A. R. Vining, and D. L. Weimer. (2001). *Cost-Benefit Analysis: Concepts and Practice*, 2nd ed. Upper Saddle River, NJ: Prentice-Hall.

Friedman L.S. (2002). *The Microeconomics of Public Policy Analysis*. Princeton, NJ: Princeton University Press, pp. 297–298.

Kingsbury, K. (2008, May 20). "The Value of a Human Life: $129,000." (See the Time Magazine website.)

Layard, R., and S. Glaister. (1994). *Cost-Benefit Analysis*, 2nd ed. Cambridge, UK: Cambridge University Press.

Wikipedia.org. (2013). "Social Discount Rate." (See the organization website.)

White House.gov. (1993). "Agency Checklist: Regulatory Impact Analysis Checklist." (See the organization website.) Note: Executive Order 12866 (September 30, 1993), 58 FR 51735 (October 4, 1993), as amended by Executive Order 13258, 67 FR 9385 (February 28, 2002) and by Executive Order 13422, 72 FR 2763 (January 23, 2007). For the complete text of the definition of "significant regulatory action," see E.O. 12866 at § 3(f). A "regulatory action" is "any substantive action by an agency (normally published in the *Federal Register*) that promulgates or is expected to lead to the promulgation of a final rule or regulation, including notices of inquiry, advance notices of proposed rulemaking, and notices of proposed rulemaking." E.O. 12866 at § 3(e).

Zerbe, R., X. Han, D. Layton, and T. Leshine. (2002). "A History of Discount Rates and Their Use by Government Agencies." Unpublished Working Paper. (See the University of Washington website.)

Key Terms

cost-effectiveness analysis Similar to cost-benefit analysis, this form of analysis does not consider societal impacts, particularly the value of human life; any analysis that fails to monetize impacts or consider human life impacts may qualify for cost-effectiveness analysis.

ex ante cost-benefit analysis A cost-benefit analysis that is conducted before the project, problem resolution, opportunity endeavor, or event.

ex post cost-benefit analysis A cost-benefit analysis that is conducted after the project, problem resolution, opportunity endeavor, or event.

future value The present-day value of a cost or benefit in the future with a known compound interest rate and period of time in years.

impact analysis An analytical approach that examines the impact a chosen decision or alternative will have on the organization, community, or society in general.

impacts A consequence to an event or decision that can be either an input or output and can be categorized and measured.

in media res cost-benefit analysis A cost-benefit analysis that is conducted during the project, problem resolution, opportunity endeavor, or event.

inputs A type of impact (asset or factor) that contributes to the development of the alternative or venture.

Kaldor-Hicks criterion A condition of Pareto efficiency that states a decision, solution, project, or alternative should be chosen if the individuals benefiting from it are able to compensate those who are made worse off by it and still be better off.

monetization Placing a money value on an impact (after it's been quantified).

Monte Carlo sensitivity analysis A form of sensitivity analysis that approximates impact values based on probabilities and also accounts for uncertainties by randomly altering impact values to determine statistically likely outcomes.

net benefits The value remaining after considering all of the benefits and deducting all of the costs.

net present value The difference between the present value of all of the benefits, less the present value of all of the costs; present value is determined by discounting the future value.

outputs A type of impact (asset or factor) that is produced as a result of an alternative or venture under consideration.

Pareto efficiency A form of efficiency in welfare microeconomics that requires that any alternative allocation in the distribution of a good or service which will make any individual better off will not make anyone else worse off.

present value The value of future cost or benefit in present day with a known social discount rate and period in years.

public good A good or service that is jointly consumed by more than one person that is nonrival (cannot diminish the good to others when used) and nonexclusive (is available to everyone without exclusion).

quality-adjusted life-years A means of determining the value of life by adjusting for the quantity of life in years and the quality of life in status that occur as a result of an alternative, decision, intervention, or venture.

regulatory impact analysis Cost-benefit analysis in government determination of regulatory policies and their impact on society.

sensitivity analysis A step in cost-benefit analysis that attempts to measure the consequences of the impact categories of various alternatives and the effect each has on the others by acknowledging the presence of uncertainty.

social discount rate The rate at which future benefits and costs should be discounted to reveal their present values.

statistical life The approximated value that an individual is willing to pay to avoid the risk of death; the economic equivalence of the social value of a human life.

time value of money The effect that time has on the value of money, such that money in the future is generally valued less than money of present day.

welfare economics A type of microeconomics that deals with equal distribution of income or goods or services to society as a whole to ensure well-being; the basis for Pareto efficiency.

CHAPTER 6 | # Impact Analysis

Objectives

After reading this chapter, the student should be able to:

6.1 Describe the application, importance, and utility of conducting an impact analysis as a stand-alone process and as an integral part of an overall analysis.

6.2 Describe the conceptual foundation and origin of impact analysis and how it can be adapted to EMS analytical approaches.

6.3 List the sequential steps in performing an impact analysis with details of the subcomponents for each step and emphasis on a multi-goal approach.

6.4 Describe the importance and meaning of primary goals, impact categories, the process of valuation, the development of alternative solution options, and political feasibility in impact analysis.

6.5 Describe the standard format of an impact analysis matrix, its relevance to a recommendation, and how it can be integrated into a final report.

Key Terms

ex ante process

ex post process

impact analysis

impact analysis matrix

impact categories

multi-goal analysis

mutually exclusive

political feasibility

primary goals

status quo alternative

WHAT WOULD YOU DO?

As the manager of a fairly large EMS agency, you are facing some important decisions stemming from the request from your board of directors to expand your coverage area to provide for a neighboring community. The neighboring community recently discovered that it cannot meet its future financial obligations to a contracted EMS organization and is in desperate need of help.

Situations such as this are not uncommon and, unfortunately, many choices made during such critical moments are based on presump-

tion, limited information at hand, and "gut" instincts. However, there is a formal approach that will help in making an informed decision.

Questions

1. If the board's request is fulfilled, how best should the expansion occur?
2. What options exist that are the most viable?
3. What are the consequences of each of the options?
4. How well will your decision be received by the community as well as by the board members?

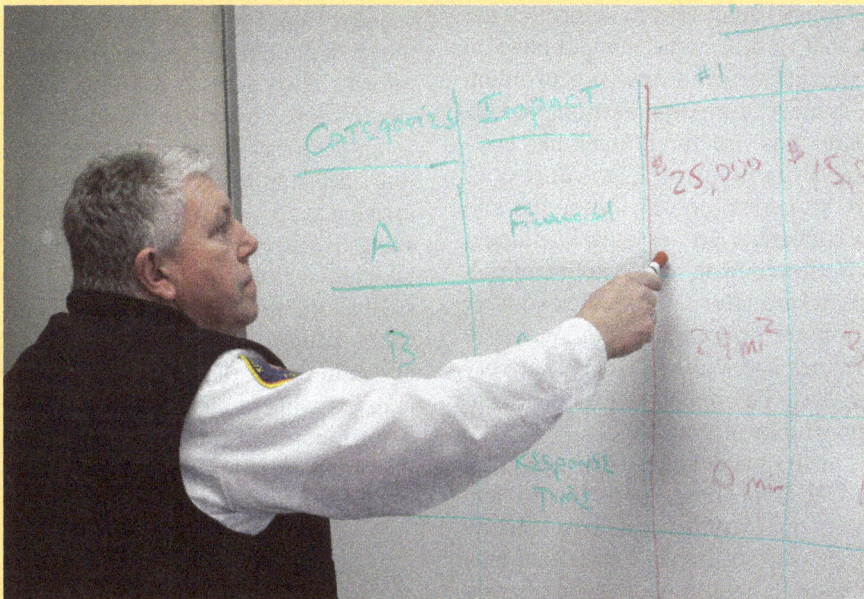

FIGURE 6.1 ■ Considering alternatives from an impact analysis.

■ INTRODUCTION ────────

In your analytical approach to problem resolution or investigating an opportunity for growth, proper identification of the

problem or opportunity is very important to set the foundation for your analysis. Having a clear understanding of the background and being familiar with the literature that deals with the specific problem is also very valuable.

Once you've begun your analysis with a firm foundation of research principles and you've analyzed the financial information and any cost-benefit analysis that you deem necessary, you may want to predict the impact your solution alternative may have on your problem, organization, system, or community. This need can be satisfied with a properly designed **impact analysis**. This chapter will describe the features and processes necessary to conduct an effective impact analysis.

THE FOUNDATION OF IMPACT ANALYSIS

The goal of impact analysis is to determine the magnitude that various impacts might have on differing alternative solutions to a problem within the context of an organization, system, or community. It is structured much like cost-benefit analysis in many aspects, but it does not require monetization of all benefits and costs to be effective. The essence of impact analysis is borrowed from the discipline of policy analysis, where alternative policies under consideration are evaluated for their overall impact (Weimer and Vining, 2011). That very same process can be applied to problem solutions or opportunity alternatives.

Impact analysis adds value to the analytical process by considering the goals of the problem resolution or opportunity endeavor and by identifying the various impacts each goal may have. This helps in determining which alternative to employ. It also helps align organizational efforts with its strategic plan and vision. Impact analysis is a very valuable component to the overall analytical process, but it actually has utility as a stand-alone analytical process in select situations. It has become very popular in federally originated programs and in industrialized and developed countries (OECD, n.d.).

When more than a few goals exist in a project or endeavor, the logical approach is a

multi-goal analysis. This is where impact analysis makes the greatest contribution. Multi-goal analysis facilitates comparisons of disparate goals. Since it is a process of comparing alternatives to the satisfaction of three or more goals, it is extremely helpful under these circumstances. As we develop our impact analysis process, you will likely appreciate the applicability of impact analysis to this approach.

THE BASIC STEPS OF CONDUCTING AN IMPACT ANALYSIS

Conducting an impact analysis consists of six consecutive steps, each having input in the subsequent step. The steps should be conducted in the prescribed order so that each preceding step informs each next step. To do otherwise may create some erroneous results that would lead to an incorrect conclusion. It is recommended that each step receive ample contemplation, as arriving at an ideal result for each step demands some insight and thought. Although there are no standardized time frames for impact analysis, it is often accomplished in a relatively short time—usually within several weeks. The scope and complexity of the project or initiative that is undergoing impact analysis are the principal determinants of the time frame. In describing the process, we'll begin with the first step: determining the **primary goals**.

DETERMINING THE PRIMARY GOALS

With each problem solution or opportunity, there exists an objective or goal that underlies its purpose. Whether it is to expand an agency's service area, acquire new equipment, develop a means of reducing operational costs, or determine the best approach to address new, unanticipated challenges to the organization, each purpose has associated goals. Most situations have more than one goal implied. For example, if expansion of

---

**Goals Associated with Expansion
of EMS Services**

Goal #1   Provide timely delivery of services

Goal #2   Provide quality care to patients

Goal #3   Minimize operational costs secondary
to expansion

Goal #4   Improve revenues from expansion

Goal #5   Gain public and political support for
expansion

FIGURE 6.2   Sample goals for service expansion.

service to a neighboring community is your organization's current challenge, then that challenge can be broken down into several goals. Figure 6.2 illustrates some examples of goals associated with service expansion.

As you can see, the objective of expanding services to the nearby communities may be associated with numerous goals. We've listed only several of them here, but you might imagine a number of others that would apply. Again, each step in the impact analysis process deserves considerable thought and contemplation. It might even be advisable to form an ad hoc committee or a focus group to brainstorm goals that might be associated with such an expansion (it's much easier to eliminate unnecessary or unimportant goals than it is to construct them after the fact).

The number of goals will vary, depending on the nature of the problem or opportunity for development. In any case, be sure to list only the primary goals and not secondary or tertiary goals. Impact analysis is a fairly intensive process and should address the larger picture and not the smaller details. If your goal selection becomes either too many or too detailed, it will cause the entire process to become cumbersome and unmanageable. Keeping the goals selection to areas of major

concern and limiting the number of goals will make the process easier to accomplish and realizable. More than six or seven goals may make the process burdensome, and ten or more goals would make it difficult to accomplish.

SELECTING IMPACT CATEGORIES

Once you've determined your primary goals, you will need to select appropriate **impact categories** for each goal. An impact category is a measurable event or outcome that results from the accomplishment of the associated goal. It should be closely tied to the goal, and its presence (or absence) or degree of presence (or degree of absence) should enable an effective assessment of achieving that goal. For example, in our first goal, we declared, "Provide timely delivery of services." This goal can be measured by a few simple means. We could preliminarily determine the geographical distances to each point in our new coverage area, taking into consideration traffic patterns and congestion, and calculate the average response times. We could also examine any preexisting data on response times from parallel services, such as fire or police, in the new coverage area.

There may be few or many impact categories for each goal. If there are many impact categories for each goal and the number of primary goals is too many, the analytical process can become unmanageable. It is more important to select all of the necessary impact categories for each goal, than it is to try to imagine every possible goal. If you can develop several essential, all-encompassing goals and select all of the meaningful impact categories for each, you will be well on your way to creating an effective impact analysis.

The time assessments discussed above are reasonable measures and they enable us to create meaningful impact categories for the first goal. It is important to note that our selection of impact categories for this first goal is based on the fact that our impact analysis will be an

**Impact Categories Associated
With Primary Goals**

Goal #1   Response time calculated from
geographic distances
Average response times from existing
public safety services

Goal #2   Crew composition
Full complement of equipment
Full complement of ALS units
Inclusion of new coverage area into
CQI performance review

Goal #3   Fixed asset costs
Crew salaries
General and administrative costs

Goal #4   Income from expanded services
Net benefits from expansion

Goal #5   Increase marketing
Assess public sentiment

FIGURE 6.3 ■ Sample impact categories for
primary goals.

ex ante **process**. If it were an *ex post* **process**, it
would be even easier to examine existing
response time data from our organization. An
ex post impact analysis may be conducted
afterward to verify our initial findings.

Some sample impact categories have been
chosen for the primary goals and are illustrated
in Figure 6.3. Although the nature and number
of impact categories will vary, it is important that
they can be measured. Unlike cost-benefit analysis, they do not need to be monetized. This is an
advantage to impact analysis because we can
value them in a variety of quantifiable terms.
Sometimes an impact category can be measured
simply by its existence. Will it exist given this
alternative or not? The answer may be a simple
yes or no. Nonetheless, that is a measurement (it
is a nominal measure) and can be recorded and
serve as a criterion for determining impact to a
particular goal or alternative.

In our example in Figure 6.3, "Full complement of equipment," "Full complement of ALS
units," and "Increase marketing" may each be
considered a nominal measure by indicating
either a yes or no response. Alternatively, we
might measure it in terms of magnitude of
increase (such as how much money will be allocated to the marketing plan). The other impact
categories will likely result in a numerical
measure, either in dollars or some other quantifiable metric. In this manner, we can compare
impacts across the list of alternative solutions.

DEVELOPING SOLUTION ALTERNATIVES

Once all of the impact categories have been
selected, we can proceed to proposing alternative solutions to our problem or opportunity
endeavor. These, too, must be thoroughly
thought out. Alternative solutions should be
viable and reasonable options. You should
avoid at all costs any sham alternatives. In this
analytical process, we are attempting to determine which solution option is the best. We
should not offer up an option we are not truly
willing to consider simply to make our preferred alternative look better or to substantiate our analysis. If there are only two
alternatives (not a preferred condition), then
considering only these two options is better
than two real options and one dummy option.

So, it is preferred that you have more than
two solution alternatives from which to choose.
Even if there are only two reasonable alternatives, you should provide at least a third alternative as a **status quo alternative**. In this
situation, you will then be comparing two viable options to doing nothing whatsoever—still
a good analytical approach. A range of solution alternatives for a good impact analysis is
between three and seven solutions.

Sometimes solution alternatives can be
quite creative and can provide not only good
solutions but also some substantive improve-
ments over the status quo. On occasion, a solu-

tion alternative is only a little different from the opposing alternatives, offering only incremental choices. However, each solution option must be **mutually exclusive**. That is, any option cannot be similar enough in nature to another one that it is merely a small variation of that option.

The opposite perspective is equally important. In addition to avoiding solution alternatives that are marginally different, avoid solution alternatives that are all inclusive and attempt to accomplish more than what the problem prescribes as necessary. Sometimes when a problem presents itself and there is leadership or public support behind solving it and funding allocated for its resolution, one may be tempted to "fix" other problems in the process. Adding this type of complexity to the impact analysis not only dilutes the process and undermines your efforts, but it also muddies the solutions. Try to keep focused on the problem that was identified and minimize any extraneous add-ons.

Another important aspect to solution alternatives is that they can be modifiable. That is, once you've progressed well into the impact analysis process, you may realize that your solution alternatives (or maybe one of the alternatives) could be improved with new or additional impact categories. That obviously will necessitate that the process be repeated, but at least it would render an improved outcome. Solution alternatives should be somewhat flexible and modifiable as the process continues.

One last important detail to keep in mind is not to choose a solution alternative *before* the process is complete. Make sure all primary goals have been identified, all impact categories have been selected, and all impacts have been suitably valued. Don't be drawn into making premature decisions—it's not until you have all the information that you should make your final decision.

In our example, we will propose three solution alternatives in our expansion plans to the neighboring communities. Our first option

is to deliver services from our existing stations in our current community. Our second option is to post units into the new coverage areas during high-volume times of the day (status system management). Our third option is to acquire, through purchase, an additional station in the new coverage area. Those three options are highlighted in Figure 6.4 as Alternative #1, Alternative #2, and Alternative #3.

PREDICTING EACH IMPACT IN TERMS OF GOAL ACHIEVEMENT

This step in the impact analysis process may be the most challenging. With the impact categories selected and your solution alternatives developed, you now need to predict how each impact will perform with each alternative. In effect, you are pulling the alternatives together to enable an effective comparison and an ultimate selection. By examining how each impact will be measured in each alternative and forecasting how that might influence the alternative outcome, you are integrating the process and refining the analytical process.

This is usually best accomplished by examining how each measurable impact performs for each goal under each solution alternative. Essentially, you will be projecting whether the impact is positive, negative, or not applicable (no effect). For example, if you wanted to know the impact performance of response times under the first goal for each of the alternatives, you could presume that response times would be higher if response originated from the existing stations. By comparison, it would be significantly improved if you were to stage units in the new coverage area during high volume times of the day and week. Finally, if stations were built or acquired within the new coverage area itself, the response times would be even more reduced.

This step is depicted in Figure 6.4 by the entries in each cell of the matrix. We have estimated impacts as positive by the plus symbol

Goal	Impact Category	Alternative #1 Existing Station	Alternative #2 Status Management	Alternative #3 New Stations
#1 Timely delivery of services	Calculated response time	--	+	++
	Existing average response times	--	+	++
#2 Quality care to patients	Crew composition	++	++	++
	Full equipment	++	++	++
	Full ALS units	+	+	++
	CQI assessment	+	+	++
#3 Reduce operational costs	Fixed asset costs	0	0	---
	Crew salaries	0	--	---
	General & administrative costs	-	--	---
#4 Improve revenue	Increased income	+	++	+++
	Net benefits	+	++	+++
#5 Gain public and political support	Increased marketing	+	+	++
	Assess public sentiment	+	++	++

FIGURE 6.4 ■ Alternative solutions for expansion.

and negative by the minus symbol. Impacts that have no performance predictions for that goal are marked with a zero. Magnitude of projected performance can also be related by the number of pluses or minuses, with a maximum of three each. Examine Figure 6.4 to gain some appreciation of the performance for each impact according to its alternative. Again, these are speculative responses, not factual results.

The logical manner in which performance is projected compels the need to understand how one would accomplish these impact measures. In other words, by forecasting performance, you are inherently implying the method as to how they are to be measured. When we selected these impact categories, we implicitly ensured that they were measurable and decided on the methodology of their measurement. The response time determination was based on known response times for given distances and comparing them to the newly established geographic distances. This

will become important in the next step when we begin valuing the impacts.

For this step, we are merely interested in a direction of performance of each impact. For some impacts, this step might suffice in determining a preferable solution alternative. However, the precision and magnitude of each impact cannot be fully appreciated until it is formally valued (measured and reported). For this reason, you are encouraged to continue in the impact analysis process to arrive at the final recommendation.

VALUING THE IMPACTS

Now that we have a good idea of the direction of performance of each impact and how we would likely measure them, we should begin the process of obtaining real numerical values for each impact measure. Obviously, this step may take some time. If we need to determine the projected response times for each alternative, we would need time to plot out the furthest points in the new coverage area, determine their distances, establish probable high-volume times and days, and estimate response time based on that data. Once collected, it would prove very valuable in our final outcome determination.

As we begin to value each impact, we may begin to realize its value as an informative source. For example, we may begin to realize that crew composition may not be a factor in any of the alternatives. Our organization's policy is to ensure high-quality delivery of services under all circumstances and that a unit does not leave the station without a full complement of crew. With that being the case, it doesn't matter what alternative solution is chosen; crew composition and quality care should be unimpeded. We may then decide to eliminate that impact category from the impact analysis. The same could be said about the full complement of advanced life support equipment.

However, by comparison, we do acknowledge that by acquiring a station in the new coverage area, we are committing to a dedicated advanced life support unit for that station, which alters the performance of that impact. Similarly, with a new station in the community, we suspect we might be more likely to focus more attention to continuous quality improvement (CQI) at that location (of course, that shouldn't change our CQI efforts, but this is illustrative only).

As we explore additional impact categories in differing goals, we recognize that some are markedly impacted by the alternatives. We will begin to see sizable differences as we record the numbers on our impact matrix from our valuation efforts. Consider the results of our findings in the final **impact analysis matrix**, illustrated in Figure 6.5.

Note that not all values in the impact analysis matrix cells are point values—some are ranges. This approach is completely acceptable as it still provides a quantifiable

means of comparison between each of the solution alternatives. In addition, now that we are formally valuing our impacts, we may discover that our predictions were not entirely accurate. Some recorded values did not bear out our predictions. By continuing the impact analysis process to the final step, we were able to avert accepting erroneous information in our final decisions.

Side Bar

Alternatives to Valuing Impacts

The valuation of most impacts typically involves microeconomic principles of supply and demand. Once the demand for an item or service is known, the price (or valuation) can be monetarily determined.

This is not the case for all impacts. Some impacts do not have a value easily placed on them (human life, polluted air, improved response times, etc.). In the past, these were regarded as intangibles and were excluded from impact analyses. However, there are ways to value these types of impacts.

One method is an indirect method known as observed behavior. In this process, the involved groups of individuals are closely observed to reveal their preferences, thus placing a value on their decisions or choices. This approach is fraught with biases (selection bias, omitted variables bias, etc.), but it can give a reasonable approximation of an impact's value.

One example of this approach is with opportunity costs (the value of something that one is willing to give up to gain something else). If you wanted to value the impact of studying for 3 hours, you could use opportunity cost as a means of valuing it. What would it take for that person to forgo studying? Go to the movies? That costs $12—now you have your impact value.

There are other methods for indirectly valuing impacts. Whatever method you employ, be sure to detail it in your impact analysis report.

Goal	Impact Category	Alternative #1 Existing Station	Alternative #2 Status Management	Alternative #3 New Stations
#1 Timely delivery of services	Calculated response time	8–14 minutes	4–14 minutes	3–10 minutes
	Existing average response times	6–12 minutes	3–12 minutes	3–12 minutes
#2 Quality care to patients	Crew composition	Paramedic and EMT	Paramedic and EMT	Paramedic and EMT
	Full Equipment	Yes	Yes	Yes
	Full ALS units	Yes, 85% of the time	Yes, 85% of the time	Yes, 95% of the time
	CQI assessment	40% of calls	40% of calls	60% of calls
#3 Reduce operational costs	Fixed asset costs	0	0	$225,000
	Crew salaries	0	$132,000 annually	$198,000 annually
	General and administrative costs	$45,000 annually	$82,000 annually	$116,000 annually
#4 Improve revenue	Increased income	$855,000 annually	$940,500 annually	$1,225,500 annually
	Net benefits	$210,000	$462,000	$612,000
#5 Gain public and political support	Increased marketing	15% increase	15% increase	25% increase
	Assess public sentiment	40% positive support	55% positive support	68% positive support

FIGURE 6.5 ■ Impact analysis matrix.

EVALUATING THE ALTERNATIVE OUTCOMES

Perhaps the easiest step, but maybe the most important, is making the final choice of solution alternatives. If all of the information indicates a clear choice, then the decision is relatively easy. What if the impact categories are very similar or seem to balance each other out? That makes the choice of alternatives much more difficult. This is where we must emphasize the most important impact categories as a means for selection. If alternatives seem somewhat similar in outcomes, but there is variance in one important impact category, then we may be able to choose the best alternative based on that one variable impact category. Of course, that implies that some risk is associated with putting that much emphasis on one impact as a means of

determining a preferred alternative. This is the principal reason why it is so important to choose impact categories that are mutually exclusive, and easily measureable, and that accurately reflect performance in the primary goals.

The other evaluative consideration that deserves attention is to consider the impact outcomes in the most important primary goals. Since the impact categories are products of the primary goals, the goals that have the greatest value or importance should drive the selection to some degree. If impact outcome variance is greater in the more important goals, then that also helps make the decision easier.

Lastly, make sure your impact valuations are valid. Any misrepresentation of any individual impact through erroneous valuation will have a multiplied influence on the impact outcomes and the ultimate decision. By systematically ensuring proper valuation of all impact categories throughout the process, you will avoid misinformation in the end of the impact analysis.

Once you have quantifiably determined the best alternative solution based on impact category valuations, you should consider just one more aspect to your decision: What is the **political feasibility** of your choice?

◼ CONSIDERING THE POLITICAL FEASIBILITY OF CHOICES——————

Imagine conducting an impact analysis with attention to detail and precision; expending considerable time and effort in determining proper goals, impact categories, and impact values; carefully analyzing the best possible solution alternative; making that recommendation; and then discovering that it is hugely unpopular with the leadership, community, or public at large. This situation is experienced by many who then regret making the recommendation at all.

When contemplating the best possible solution alternative, you should also consider the political feasibility of the solution. If the solution is likely to meet substantive resistance from stakeholders, especially decision makers and officials, then making the recommendation without qualifications could be disastrous. For this reason, it is important to value each alternative with some measure of political feasibility. It needn't be a formal measure, such as a survey or interview, but being as close to the nature of the problem as you will likely be, you should have an accurate appreciation of the sentiments of those it will affect or those who will be responsible for the ultimate decision. Consider the consequences of each alternative when making your selection.

This can also be mitigated by making clear the consequences of each alternative in your recommendation and clarifying the

political fallout of each alternative. When making the formal recommendations, be sure to cite any political concerns you might suspect exist so that the decision makers can be fully informed up front.

◼ MAKING THE RECOMMENDATION——————

Now that all of the analytical process is complete and a choice has been made of the alternative solutions, a formal recommendation should be offered to the decision makers or stakeholders of the organization. Obviously, if the decision maker is you, this step is unnecessary.

The recommendation should be developed in written form and should consist of all of the relevant elements. If the impact analysis is part of a larger analytical approach (as it often is), the recommendation should be part of the overall report. If the impact analysis stands alone, a report should be written making the recommendations based on findings and political feasibility.

The stand-alone impact analysis report should consist of each of the following:

+ A description of the problem or opportunity that details what the problem is, why it is a problem, and what potential consequence the problem may create
+ Some background on the problem, a contributory history, or a summary of the political landscape that surrounds the problem
+ Any literature search information that might help inform the problem or opportunity, such that it can support and underscore the recommendation that is made and help make the decision easier and have greater credibility
+ A description of the process or methodology of the selection of the primary goals, the impact categories, and the solution alternative designs (You may also want to include the methods employed in the valuation of each of the impacts.)

* The results of the impact analysis (Often this is best displayed in an impact analysis matrix, much like the one in Figure 6.5, with explanation and details in the textual portion of the report.)
* The rationales and logic behind the selection of the preferred solution alternative and projection of outcomes associated with that selection (This should include both positive and negative consequences as well as any political impacts.)
* A summary of any referential information used in the analysis

This report needn't be lengthy, but it should be inclusive of the preceding information. Simple problems or opportunities typically generate smaller impact analyses, whereas complex problems can result in substantive reports with multiple appendices and supportive documents. In the end, the report is a representation of all of your efforts, so it should appear professional, well organized, and legible without grammatical and composition errors, and it should reach a reasonable conclusion. Some reports are bound, but most are simply printed and collated with the pages secured in a binder or folder.

Best Practices

Regulatory Impact Analysis at the Federal Level

In September 2003, the Office of Management and Budget of the White House issued Circular A-004 on the Best Practices guidelines for Regulatory Impact Analysis (RIA). This circular revised the previous version issued in 1996 and 2000. The circular addresses the guidelines necessary for all federal agencies to follow with regard to RIAs under the Regulatory Right-to-Know Act.

The regulatory impact analysis is a tool to measure and evaluate the likely consequences of rules on an industry or society as a whole. It examines alternatives that are under consideration for developing regulations and are intended to disclose whether or not the benefits of a proposed rule or regulation is likely to justify the costs associated with it and to disclose which of the alternatives is most cost effective. Cost-benefit analysis is the fundamental tool within regulatory impact analysis.

A product of these regulatory laws and implementation guidelines is the adoption of RIAs by the United States Environmental Protection Agency (EPA) in the development of national air pollution regulations. An example of the Best Practices Guidelines is the EPA's implementation of an RIA in June 2010 for short-term sulfur dioxide (SO_2) National Ambient Air Quality Standards (NAAQS). Using the current air monitoring systems, the objective of the RIA in this application was to provide the public with an estimate of the costs and benefits of attaining new sulfur dioxide air quality standards, while maintaining compliance with the new Executive Order 12866, which generated the OMB Circular A-004.

In current practice, all federal agencies are expected to abide by the new regulatory impact analysis guidelines for every regulation and policy that may have a significant impact on industry, quality of life, and society in general. This national standard for federal agencies has set higher levels of performance benchmarks for all other industries, private or public. It is reasonable to expect the delivery of EMS to be included in this elevated standard.

For more information on the EPA's regulatory impact analysis implementations, see: www.epa.gov/ttnecas1/ria.html. For more information on the OMB's guidelines for RIAs in response to Executive Order 12866, see the White House website.

CHAPTER REVIEW

Summary

Conducting an impact analysis is often a very useful tool in the analytical approach to EMS or any other discipline. It offers a unique perspective on problems or opportunities and their potential solutions or endeavors. The impact analysis provides us with a different view of solutions by examining what consequences may occur as a result of their implementation. Like any analytical approach, impact analysis is not foolproof or terminal in its findings, but rather another instrument in the overall analytical approach intending to better inform us.

The process is straight forward. Once the problem has been properly identified and an adequate background established, the impact analysis approach begins with establishing primary goals expected from the solution. Then, appropriate impact categories are identified with measureable capacities and goal

relevance. The potential solutions to the problem should be designed based on satisfaction of the impacts and primary goals. At this stage a projection or forecast of the impact categories is made, followed by an actual valuation of each of the impacts. This information is then entered into an impact analysis matrix where illustration of the best alternative is likely. The chosen alternative is then recommended in a formal written report.

Analytical approaches often contain an impact analysis when they are complete in their scope of analysis, but impact analysis can remain a stand-alone analysis in select circumstances. When integrated into a broad analysis, impact analysis provides a unique perspective into the solutions or opportunities that no other approach can provide. It is a very useful adaption from its origin in policy analysis.

WHAT WOULD YOU DO? Reflection

Understanding the process behind impact analysis will enable you to better formulate viable options and sort out the alternatives more effectively. There is an investment of time and effort, but the outcome is likely to be invaluable. Thinking about what goals need to be accomplished and what impacts may occur in the pursuit of those goals will help immensely in clarifying the problem. As you gather information and begin to value each impact category, the picture becomes more clear and the choices become increasingly evident.

Once you've completed your impact analysis, you can make a reasonably informed choice. Now, you must consider what politi-

cal impact this recommendation might have. After examining and contemplating the political feasibility of each alternative under consideration, you arrive at the best choice. You take the time to draft a comprehensive document that reports your recommendation, complete with references, data charts, and an impact analysis matrix, and present it to your board of directors. After reviewing your report, they unanimously agree with your recommendation. Without question, the detail of your report and the completeness of your investigation facilitated their decision with little deliberation. Your recommendation was a complete success.

Review Questions

1. How does impact analysis add to the entire analytical approach?
2. Why should the steps of impact analysis be performed in their specified order?
3. Is it better to have many goals, or to have only several encompassing goals? And, how many alternative solutions should you propose for comparison?
4. What is a status quo alternative and what value does it have?
5. What is a mutually exclusive alternative and why is it important?
6. Why is the step of predicting impact outcomes in terms of goal achievement important in the impact analysis process?
7. How is it acceptable that impact categories needn't be monetized?
8. What are the elements of an impact analysis matrix and why is this important?
9. Why should political feasibility be considered before the final recommendation is made in impact analysis?
10. How should the results of an impact analysis be presented?

References

Boardman, A. E., D. H. Greenberg, A. R. Vining, and D. L. Weimer. (2011). *Cost-Benefit Analysis: Concepts and Practice*, 4th ed. Upper Saddle River, NJ: Prentice Hall.

OECD. (n.d.). "Regulatory Impact Analysis." (See the organization website.)

Weimer, D. L., and A. R. Vining. (2011). *Policy Analysis*, 5th ed. Upper Saddle River, NJ: Pearson, pp. 340–382.

Key Terms

ex ante **process** In impact analysis, when the analytical process occurs before the problem is resolved, opportunity is begun, or a project is launched.

ex post **process** In impact analysis, when the analytical process occurs after the problem is resolved, opportunity is begun, or a project is launched as a means of evaluating success.

impact analysis An analytical process adopted from policy analysis that enables a systematic assessment of alternative solutions to a problem on the basis of goals and impacts each alternative has on each goal through valuation of impact outcomes.

impact analysis matrix An illustrative table that details each of the primary goals and their associated impact categories against each of the problem solution alternatives; summarizing the impact analysis in a table format.

impact categories Ways that the primary goals can be measured; occurrences or events that result from the accomplishment of the primary goals.

multi-goal analysis The process of examining a problem or opportunity by identifying the goals necessary for its resolution and comparing the impacts that occur for each goal.

mutually exclusive In impact analysis, a condition of problem alternatives whereby each solution alternative is unique from the other and not a variation of one theme.

political feasibility The acceptability of a proposed solution to stakeholders and decision makers regardless of its effectiveness to resolve the problem.

primary goals The identified purposes to be accomplished by each alternative solution; what the resolution hopes to achieve.

status quo alternative In impact analysis, the problem solution alternative that does nothing, but keeps the situation the same; a means of comparative analysis by examining impact categories against the current situation.

Feasibility Analysis

Objectives

After reading this chapter, the student should be able to:

7.1 Demonstrate an understanding of the applicability and typical forms of feasibility analysis as a solitary application and as an element in a comprehensive analytical approach.

7.2 Demonstrate an understanding of the benefits and limitations of feasibility analysis and the two evaluative goals of cost and value.

7.3 Describe the relationships between feasibility analysis and that of financial analysis and cost-benefit analysis in the overall analytical approach.

7.4 Define economic feasibility, technical feasibility, and operational feasibility, and describe their constituent components, how they are applied, and how they relate to other forms of analysis.

7.5 Describe concept testing, receptivity testing, and legal feasibility analysis, their differences, and their applicability in feasibility studies.

7.6 Demonstrate an understanding of the concepts of the scope of operations and resource sufficiency and how they apply to feasibility analysis, their benefits, and limitations.

7.7 Demonstrate an understanding of SWOT analysis, GAP analysis, and force field analysis, how they apply to feasibility analysis, and their benefits and limitations.

Key Terms

concept testing
cost-benefit analysis
costs
economic feasibility
external environment
feasibility study
financial analysis

force field analysis
gap analysis
intangible
internal environment
legal feasibility
operational feasibility
receptivity testing

resource sufficiency
scope of operations
SWOT analysis
technical feasibility
value

WHAT WOULD YOU DO?

Crews have been approaching you about expanding services to include community paramedic care. As the organization's operational officer, you can appreciate the value this endeavor might bring to the community and to the financial well-being of your organization. Your greatest concerns are the financial outlay, the risk of this endeavor, and whether or not the local community would embrace it.

1. How can you go about investigating the likely outcomes of these concerns?
2. Should you proceed with this new service?
3. The crews seem to be in favor, and the remainder of the management team endorses this initiative as well. What should you do?

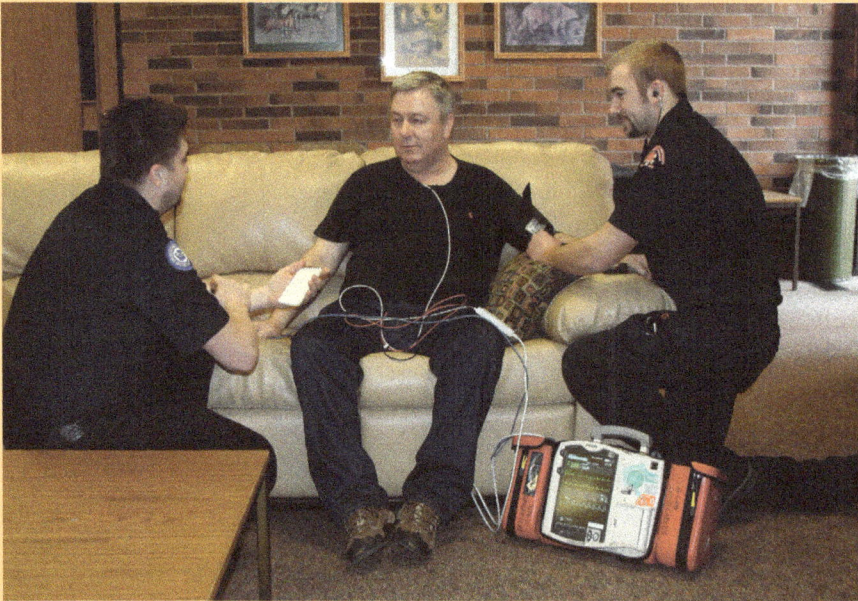

FIGURE 7.1 ■ Community-oriented primary health care.

■ INTRODUCTION

Feasibility analysis, sometimes referred to as a **feasibility study**, attempts to determine whether or not to proceed with a business venture or project. It is often employed as a singular analysis of a "go" or "no go" decision. Many entrepreneurial companies explore new product lines or venture into diverse processes by first conducting feasibility studies.

In its simplest version, a feasibility study is a contemplative consideration as to whether or not to proceed with an idea or desire. In its most general form, it is an evaluative process that examines an organization's financial and operational resources along with the market's acceptance of a new endeavor. The information that a feasibility analysis provides as a decision-making instrument is only as reliable and accurate as the information used to develop it. For this reason, feasibility studies should either not be relied on solely, or should employ the many aspects of analysis to render a reliable and accurate recommendation.

▓ FEASIBILITY ANALYSIS————

Feasibility analysis is a preliminary evaluative process used to determine if an idea or business venture is worth pursuing. Often, this centers on financial matters and market concerns. A thorough analytical approach should be more inclusive than just those two elements, but in some instances it is all that is necessary. Take, for example, a product company that maintains a close watch on its financial performance, market trends, customer feedback, quality improvement processes, and resource utilization. With this level of control, the consideration to venture into a new product line may only require a feasibility analysis with little risk of loss. It is when feasibility analysis is used to determine the disposition of a major investment or project without a foundation of analysis that it may be misleading.

For the most part, feasibility analyses are a part of a larger analytical approach that aids in determining whether or not an idea, opportunity for growth, or a major investment in a problem resolution is a viable option. Generally, the outcomes are that the analysis was done and indicated that it was reasonable to proceed, or it was done and it is not reasonable to proceed. Feasibility analyses typically do not provide a scaled recommendation or a magnitude of confidence relative to a decision to proceed. It's either "probably okay" or it's "probably not okay" to proceed. Again, feasibility analyses are very useful, but they have their greatest value when combined with other analytical approaches in important decision making.

TYPICAL APPLICATIONS OUTSIDE OF EMS

Probably the greatest applicability of feasibility analysis outside of EMS is in new business ventures and the development of new product lines in production companies. Other applications make it useful in the business arena.

When an existing business's leadership is interested in expansion, it may consider a feasibility study as to the financial rewards the expansion might bring as well as the receptivity by the consumer. A feasibility study can be designed to evaluate those aspects of the expansion. A similar approach can be made when a business is considering taking over another business. This type of situation may also occur in EMS when an existing agency is asked to provide coverage for (or is contemplating covering) an area currently serviced by a fledgling agency.

If a production company is interested in a new product line, the financial and production resources may be well known by the management, but receptivity by the consumer may be in question—that is, "How popular will the new product be?" Feasibility studies can help illuminate that aspect of the new venture. It is more than just a market analysis as it considers the company's business structure and capacities as well.

Feasibility analysis is conducted not only by private industry but also by government agencies. Many government initiatives are preceded by a feasibility study to determine their value and longevity of purpose. Feasibility analysis can take many forms and has many applications in both the private and public sectors.

One final purpose for conducting a feasibility study is not for the financial assessment, or even the market analysis, but to determine the company's ability to engage in the new project or business initiative. Notice that this is not motivated by the company's capacity to perform to the new demands of the proposed initiative but, rather, the *ability* to perform in response to them. Sometimes it is prudent to evaluate management's ability to engage in new activity. Conducting a feasibility analysis can offer some perspective on the demands placed on management by these new initiatives outside of what was anticipated. This is a unique benefit that feasibility analysis can provide, which may prove to be useful application to EMS.

TWO EVALUATIVE GOALS OF FEASIBILITY ANALYSIS

For the most part, feasibility analysis attempts to evaluate two important aspects of the organization when considering whether or not to pursue a new idea or initiative. They are the **costs** imposed on the organization and the **value** of the new venture or initiative. There are other reasons to conduct a feasibility study, but cost and value are the foremost reasons and are common to most studies.

Cost

Aside from its traditional meaning of the value assigned to the production of a product or the delivery of a service in the context of doing business, the term *cost* can also have a slightly different meaning in an economic sense. It can be used as a metric that results from a process or as a differential in decision making. In this context, cost is an important parameter in the feasibility analysis to determine whether a project, initiative, or investment is viable and worthy of pursuit. Most important decisions center on the financial impacts of that decision. As such, an adequate financial analysis is often necessary and may become part of the feasibility analysis.

Value

Value, in this context, goes beyond the simple monetary value of the product or service venture but, instead, the value this initiative brings to the organization. It might be increased sales or services, improved productivity, boosted employee morale, improved consumer satisfaction, or all of these. The value aspect in feasibility analysis often involves an **intangible** quality, as in customer appreciation or an improved *esprit de corps* of the company. When an agency takes a risk and pursues a new venture and that effort pays huge dividends, the benefit the organization receives from that pursuit can be almost immeasurable. Assessing and determining the value of a venture is not quite so easy. It does involve some monetary assessment, particularly in cost-benefit analysis, but it may also include a nonmonetary assessment. Both should be considered in all feasibility analyses.

APPLICATION OF FEASIBILITY ANALYSIS IN EMS

Much like other businesses, EMS professionals can apply feasibility analysis as a stand-alone analytical element. However, to ensure fully reliable information that provides a high level of validity in its recommendation for a decision, feasibility analysis should be part of an overall analytical approach.

The utility for feasibility studies in EMS is not as dissimilar as it is for traditional business applications: expansion or consolidation initiatives, new services to clients, problem resolutions, evaluations for new projects, or sizable investments in property, plant, or equipment. Many of the challenges facing an EMS agency can be informed by first conducting a feasibility analysis—not just to assess cost and value of the venture but viability as well.

For example, if an EMS agency is contemplating providing wheelchair services and nonemergent public assistance transport services, it might be well served to conduct a feasibility analysis before investing money in the equipment. Can the organization handle the additional financial burden? Will the community support this new venture (not just in utilization but also in political support)? This

situation, and many others, may be better informed by a feasibility analysis, particularly as a component of an overall analysis.

Choosing to do a feasibility analysis requires a commitment of resources and solidarity among the leadership to acknowledge the findings. A feasibility study has limited value if it is only partially implemented. Furthermore, what is the benefit of conducting a feasibility study if the results will be ignored? Or, how valuable is the feasibility analysis results if they are not embraced by all members of the management team? There must be unity in support of conducting such analyses and an agreement to abide by its results (provided the analysis is conducted properly).

Now that we've decided to proceed with the feasibility analysis and management is fully behind it, how do we proceed? What type of feasibility analysis needs to be completed? These are the subjects of the following sections.

TYPES OF FEASIBILITY ANALYSES

To properly regard feasibility analysis, one must consider the various types of studies that fall under this category. These different types of feasibility analyses result from the fact that most feasibility studies are conducted independently of any other analyses and often in isolation. Organizations that are considering a new venture, project, or expansion of services may first regard feasibility studies as self-sufficient. However, as mentioned at the onset of this chapter, deriving a fully informative analysis may require additional components to an overall analytical approach. Nonetheless, we will examine the different types of feasibility analyses even though we are more likely to include feasibility analysis as part of a larger analytical process.

The general types of feasibility analyses are economic, technical, legal, and operational. Each will be discussed separately.

ECONOMIC FEASIBILITY

Economic feasibility analysis is a process of assessing the financial prudence of an organization in its pursuit of a new venture or expansion. This type of analysis is a direct descendant from the *cost* goal of feasibility analysis. It focuses on the economic expenditure and revenues of a project, venture, expansion, project, or investment. Elemental components of this form of feasibility analysis are **financial analysis** and **cost-benefit analysis**.

Financial Analysis

Financial analysis is a methodical assessment of the organization's financial performance with regard to its assets and expenditures. These performances are often revealed in the organization's financial statements: the balance sheet, income statement, cash flow statement, and any pro forma statements that are available. This level of analysis is critical and fairly complex.

If a feasibility study is being conducted as part of an overall analytical approach that already includes a financial analysis component, then including it in the feasibility analysis is redundant and unnecessary. Our approach will be comprehensive and inclusive and will assume a financial analysis will be part of the overall analytical approach.

Cost-Benefit Analysis

In addition to the financial analysis section, a cost-benefit analysis is critical to the economic feasibility study. Since feasibility analyses focus on decisions as to whether or not to proceed with an initiative or venture based on its value to the organization, a cost-benefit analysis is germane to that concept. It is reasonable to assume that a thorough cost-benefit analysis will be completed as part of the overall analytical approach. If it is completed as part of the overall analytical approach, it would be unnecessary to repeat it in the feasibility study.

TECHNICAL FEASIBILITY

Technical feasibility raises this question: "Can the organization actually perform the new initiative or project?" The assessment focus here is on the *functional ability* of the organization to meet the production or service demands for the new initiative. Some initiatives are simply outside the scope of performance of an organization. If so, either the organization should abandon the idea or expand capabilities to include the new initiative. The only way to determine this is to conduct a technical feasibility analysis.

An example of technical feasibility analysis in EMS might be the consideration of initiating community paramedicine as part of the organization's complement of services. Although community paramedic services entail a different set of skills and objectives than the traditional role of paramedic, it still remains within the scope of performance of most paramedic systems. Perhaps some additional education and directives may be necessary, but it is not unrealistic to expect an EMS agency to extend services to include community paramedical services. This dimension represents a technical feasibility determination. Much of this form of feasibility analysis is qualitative in nature and does not require a detailed analysis. Simply examining the scopes of practice between traditional paramedic care and community paramedic care may suffice in satisfying the technical feasibility analysis.

Seeking outside perspectives from medical authorities and municipal authorities, as well as conducting literature searches, can often supplement the technical feasibility analysis. This aspect of technical feasibility is not structurally firm and is flexible in its adaptability to meet the specific needs of the organization.

Evaluating Whether the Service is Within the Scope of Delivery

In determining whether or not the proposed service is within the scope of the delivery of services, the analysis may be simple. Using the example of considering the addition of a community paramedicine service, it may be as simple as examining the curricula of both traditional and community paramedic practices and deciding if the new venture is a reasonable extension of services. It might be somewhat more complex, requiring some additional insight. To make a determination, two approaches are recommended: concept testing and receptivity testing

Concept Testing. Before launching a project, problem resolution, or new venture, leadership in the organization needs to be certain the idea will be well received by the consumers, the public, and any stakeholders. In essence, there should be a preliminary testing of the idea or concept. This is the foundational basis for **concept testing**: to test an idea before it's launched.

In production environments, this is usually accomplished by making a prototype available to consumers and then gauging their response to it. In service industries like EMS, this can be accomplished by extending the new service, project, initiative, or venture into a sample population that is representative of the targeted clientele. This might mean extending services to a subsection of the neighboring community, requesting a demonstration from the vendor of the new piece of equipment for the EMS providers, or reviewing the curriculum of community paramedicine with the paramedical staff.

At times, a less pragmatic approach can be made that is somewhat cursory and less revealing. The idea or concept could be floated to specific officials or stakeholders to judge their response or solicit their endorsement before formally launching the initiative. In this manner, less public dissemination of information is maintained to protect proprietary interests, while still assessing the idea's receptivity. This approach is somewhat analogous to tabletop exercises in disaster planning whereby conceptual methodology trials are conducted but the actual execution of the plan is not.

If confidentiality of the concept is not a concern, then initiatives can be tested through flyers, brochures, telephonic or Web-based surveys, community-based focus groups, or even through social media. In this manner, feedback can be sought without a substantive investment of resources. Many business ventures are put through trials on the Internet before they receive approval for a full implementation. Perhaps a simple electronic survey sent to a neighboring community asking about public sentiment regarding your organization's expansion could save a lot of time and money spent on an unnecessary expansion. Surveying other EMS organizations across the country about their satisfaction with a particular piece of equipment might help make a purchasing decision much easier. These are forms of concept testing in that they determine, for the organization, the prudence of proceeding with the concept or initiative.

Usability or Receptivity Testing. Usability or **receptivity testing** is very similar in design and purpose to concept testing, except the actual service (or product) is deployed. In receptivity testing, either the targeted public receives the proposed service on a limited basis for a preliminary evaluation or the product under consideration for purchase is used by the EMS providers to assess usability. Some manufacturers will permit their product to be used on a trial basis for a predetermined period to allow the users an opportunity to evaluate the product and gain familiarity. If the product has a history of considerable quality and customer satisfaction, this maneuver is often to the vendor's benefit in the long run.

A similar approach could be made with extending a new service. In the community paramedic venture example, only a few paramedics may be sent to obtain the education at that level of certification. With the few paramedics trained, the initiative could be tested for receptivity or applicability in select service areas. If the concept is well received and deemed effective, then additional personnel can be trained in community paramedic care.

Alternatively, services could be extended to a subsection of the community intended for inclusion in your service area to test their satisfaction with your delivery of services while simultaneously assessing the financial, operational, and personnel impact this expansion might have on your organization. Usability or receptivity testing can take many forms and range from the most superficial to a protracted and in-depth analysis. In almost all cases, it should be well planned with a finite time line for trial evaluation.

Technical feasibility analysis has many benefits. It can help prevent unnecessary start-ups that would draw considerable resources. It can help an organization define exactly what type and level of service a community may need. It can facilitate selection of ideal equipment and organizational needs. In addition, it can help identify the best manner of delivery with regard to time and design of newly developed services.

LEGAL FEASIBILITY

Identifying financial and value-driven factors in an organization's pursuit of an initiative or growth potential is important, but it may be halted if the implementation is curtailed by legal or regulatory restrictions. Before any venture or initiative is launched, an investigation into the **legal feasibility** is essential.

Is the venture or initiative permissible under current municipal ordinances, state laws, and federal guidelines? There must be an investigation into the potential restrictions imbued by practice guidelines, regulations, and legal constraints. This process will most often demand the services of an attorney, but many federal and state mandates and regulations can be revealed through Internet sources and state offices of EMS.

Most EMS organizations are already quite familiar with their local municipal statutes, state guidelines, and federal directives. Even regulatory restrictions can be quite transparent when the proper documents are examined closely. However, expanding services into neighboring communities or across state borders can invoke new guidelines and regulatory restrictions. It is prudent to investigate these restrictions before venturing forth.

Many EMS organizations retain legal solicitors for these reasons, and many more. Reliable legal resources are incredibly important when considering a new venture, expansion, acquisition, or organizational change. Most major purchases, investments, and problem solutions require little legal consultation. Situations should be evaluated on a case-by-case basis.

OPERATIONAL FEASIBILITY

Operational feasibility is the analytical process of determining if an initiative or venture can be executed by an organization given its current operational capacity and delivery model. It examines the conformity of the venture with the organization's current scope of operations, and it evaluates the adequacy of resources for its implementation. It also evaluates whether the initiative aligns with the organization's mission, vision, and long-term strategic plan. Operational feasibility is a very important analysis to conduct on any significant venture.

Management within most organizations is often inclined to believe that expanding operations to accommodate a new initiative, expansion, or service line is well within its capabilities. However, unless an objective analysis on the operational feasibility is conducted, the venture may prove to be overwhelming and disastrous if implemented. Not only could it produce unwarranted financial drain on an organization and some depletion of resources, but it could also cause irrevocable damage to the agency's public image.

It must be acknowledged that financial and cost-benefit analyses remain integral in determining operational capacity; however, there are other logistic concerns as well. The operational feasibility analysis will address those concerns outside of the financial and cost-benefit focus.

Scope of Operations

In this aspect of operational analysis, the feasibility of committing current operations to meet the demands of the new initiative is assessed. Most new initiatives cannot be adequately addressed without some modification or enhancement of operations—whether it is training and education, a change in operational processes and procedures, or a redeployment of resources within a different structure.

The **scope of operations** entails not only capacity of services and efficient delivery of services, but also practice standards, adherence to performance benchmarks, and compliance with organizational goals. In EMS, the concept of *scope* is just slightly different from most business models. In EMS, like most businesses, scope can mean the extent that operational services are delivered, such as coverage areas, response times, types of services delivered, and contractual service commitments. However, given its medical emphasis, scope in EMS can also mean the extent of medical services, such

as medical procedures, treatment protocols, drug formularies, and practice standards. This additional dimension adds complexity to the assessment of the scope of operations.

When a new initiative or venture is under consideration, the operational scope and practice scope of the organization must be assessed for congruency. The example offered previously of initiating community paramedic services impacts both operational aspects of the organization and the practice aspect in the delivery of care. Scope of operations is an important element of the operational feasibility analysis.

Resource Sufficiency

Resource sufficiency determination has many similarities to the financial analysis component in the economic feasibility assessment; it examines the adequacy of assets that the organization has to launch the initiative. The difference here is that the assessment is not of a monetary nature but, rather, of a physical inventory nature. The determination is to estimate the type and amount of resources necessary to launch and support the new initiative or venture. What resources need to be acquired above and beyond what currently exists?

Determining resource needs is a matter of projecting material and workforce needs for the initiative and comparing that to the current pool of resources. In almost all cases, a new initiative or venture will demand an increase in resources to support it. The financial analysis component of the economic feasibility will help determine the financial capacity to acquire the additional resources, and resource assessment will determine what resources are necessary. A simple resource list tied to the operational demands of the initiative often is sufficient. The list may then be compiled and organized into a spreadsheet so that increases in operational demand will result in a proportional increase in resource amounts. Figure 7.2 illustrates an abbreviated

Resource Demands from Incremental Expansion of Operations

	Resource Description	Current Allocation	Allocation with 10% Increase Operations	Allocation with 20% Increase Operations
1	Ambulances (units)	2	2	3
2	Staff-EMTs (FTEs)	6	6	9
3	Staff-Paramedics (FTEs)	4	4	6
4	Staff- Clerical/ Administrative (FTEs)	3	3.1	3.3
5	Durable Equipment Supply ($)	$45,000	$72,000	155,000
6	Soft Supplies ($)	$62,000	$68,200	$74,400
7	Fleet Maintenance (hours)	10/week	10/week	15/week
8	Fuel ($)	$720/week	$800/week	$1,080/week

FIGURE 7.2 Determining resource sufficiency in operational demands.

version of the resource assessment spreadsheet for a simple expansion of services.

SWOT Analysis

SWOT analysis is a means to determine an organization's position within its industry as a part of strategic planning. (The acronym SWOT stands for *Strengths, Weaknesses, Opportunities,* and *Threats.*) Despite its origin in strategic planning, SWOT analysis has also gained relevance in feasibility analysis. SWOT analysis has great applicability in operational feasibility analysis as it helps to inform the organization's operational capabilities from an internal perspective as well as in comparison to its competitors. Other analytical approaches from other disciplines also have adaptability to feasibility analysis, but SWOT analysis is the most commonly applied.

SWOT analysis begins with a candid assessment of the organization's **internal environment**: its strengths and weaknesses. This process is not only subjective and qualitative in nature; it also relies on factual data. To begin the first step in SWOT analysis, information

must be gathered relating to the organization's performance against established national and practice benchmarks, community demographics (including projected call volumes), current and future revenue streams, technology status (state-of-the-art equipment and equipment needs), staffing patterns, and lost calls, response times, and patient satisfaction surveys. Additional types of data may be useful depending on what the organization deems important and what it monitors.

From this data, a panel of diversified participants from within the organization examines the information and identifies the most positive attributes of the organization, as well as the most challenged characteristics. They are then categorized into either strengths or weaknesses (areas in need of improvement). Strengths are generally those aspects that are viewed as well established, are associated with outstanding performance, or are unique attributes that distinguish the organization from other similar organizations.

The weaknesses are any aspects of the organization that demand some level of improvement. They may be deficient areas in quality of care or burdened with excessive expense within the operational scope of delivery of services, outdated equipment, a growing response time average, and especially poor morale among personnel. Such weaknesses often have gone unnoticed or been ignored. Now that SWOT analysis has drawn attention to them, the appropriate corrective action is warranted. A focused analysis of each of the weaknesses may disclose an underlying cause that can be effectively resolved and may result in improvement of several areas of weakness. Many instances of discovered weaknesses are easily remediated with education and training, such as leadership education, strategic planning courses, or instruction in interpreting financial statements. The opportunities for improving management and leadership practices in EMS continue to grow in both traditional classrooms and online courses.

Once the internal assessments of the organization are complete, attention is then directed outward to the **external environment**. In SWOT analysis, the external environment centers on opportunities and threats. Opportunities are any initiatives or ventures that may prove to be beneficial to the organization. This is where the mind is free to wander and consider the loftiest opportunities, for they can be pared down to more realistic ones later. When applying SWOT analysis to feasibility analysis, this is also where the initiative or opportunity for growth of interest should be included. By virtue of its inclusion here, you will be comparing it to other opportunities and initiatives and contrasting it with the internal environment of the organization (strengths and weaknesses) as well as the external threats. In doing so, you will have a much better perspective of your proposed initiative.

The *threats* part of SWOT analysis refers to the *potential* events or circumstances that might pose a problem for the organization in the future. They may be very real or simply perceived. Nonetheless, they deserve mention in the threats category. Threats can materialize as almost anything that has potential to damage the organization, such as the belief that a new for-profit EMS agency is moving into your coverage area and will be competing for patients; changes in reimbursement profiles for Medicare and Medicaid recipients; and even anticipation of a downturn in the economy. Virtually anything can be included under the category of threats, but all should be truly possible and not simply feared.

Once all of the categorical information is gathered, it can then be summarized into a SWOT matrix as illustrated in Figure 7.3. By constructing a SWOT matrix, you can more easily compare and appreciate each of the categorical elements and decide on your initiative's feasibility with greater confidence. SWOT analysis helps to put the organization's strategic position into perspective relative to the initiative or venture of your intended pursuit.

An additional analysis that can be performed from your SWOT analysis is a **gap analysis**. A gap analysis examines the differences (or gaps) between the organization's internal and external environments. In effect, you are looking at the strengths and weaknesses and identifying any weaknesses that may eventually lead to a loss of opportunity or a threat from the external environment. For example, if your SWOT analysis revealed that the medical equipment on the ambulances is somewhat out of date and does not represent new technology, then advancing the organization into a new service line (such as community paramedic) would be difficult or problematic. This external opportunity (community paramedic) is nullified by the existing weakness (outdated equipment) and was identified by a gap analysis.

Force Field Analysis. There is one other analytical process that you may consider once the SWOT analysis is complete: a **force field analysis**. A force field analysis is the process of taking what was learned in your SWOT analysis and attempting to determine the driving

	Facilitates Initiative	Impedes Initiative
Internal Environment	**Strengths** • Strong leadership • Talented personnel • New equipment • Progressive philosophy • Financial liquidity	**Weaknesses** • Demanding call volume • No recent growth • Services priced too low • Payer mix worsening • High turnover of staff
External Environment	**Opportunities** • New service line (community paramedic) • New paramedic education program in area • Neighboring communities interest in services	**Threats** • New EMS agency considering entry into market • Economic downturn in local communities • Vendor costs increased

FIGURE 7.3 ■ Sample SWOT matrix.

forces behind both potential successes and potential failures. The forces that are driving successes are termed *facilitative forces*, and those that contribute toward potential failure are termed *restrictive forces*.

To properly develop a force field analysis, you must consider the organization's mission, vision, goals, and needs. In addition, you should look outside of your organization to acknowledge developing trends or contemporary ideas within the profession. These considerations help to organize your force field analysis into the categories of potential successes or failures. An example of a force field analysis is illustrated in Figure 7.4.

INCLUDING THE FEASIBILITY ANALYSIS INTO THE OVERALL ANALYTICAL APPROACH

As mentioned, feasibility analysis can be a stand-alone approach, or it can be part of a larger, overall analysis. When conducted as a separate analysis, the results are often reported in a consolidated document that depicts all of the findings in a systematic format. The sections would follow the elements as outlined in this chapter.

If the feasibility analysis is part of a larger analytical approach, it becomes one part of a comprehensive and summative analysis. The general design would include sections on problem identification, background, literature details, investigative research methodologies and findings, financial and cost-benefit analyses (which become integral to the feasibility analysis component), impact analysis, feasibility analysis, and the general conclusions and recommendations of the analysis. When compiled, each element of the analysis is used to inform other elements and all contribute to the terminal conclusions and recommendations. Like any other comprehensive process, this analysis should be concise, systematic, and accurate.

An integrative analysis as proposed here will prove to be significantly more informative than any singular analysis or component of analysis. Each element is unique in its examination of the problem or opportunity and, as such, provides uniquely valuable information toward the best decisions.

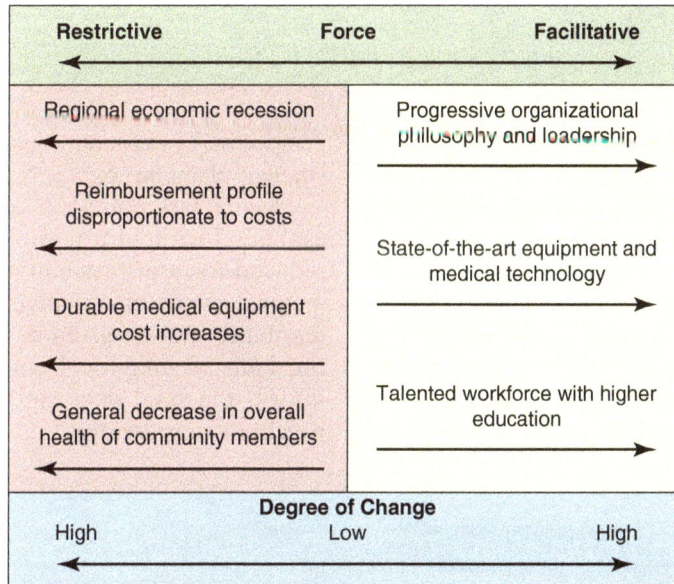

FIGURE 7.4 Sample force field analysis.

Best Practices

Feasibility Study on Surveillance of Illness and Injury in the EMS Workforce

The National Highway Traffic Safety Administration conducted a feasibility study in 2007 to determine whether an effective illness and injury surveillance of the EMS workforce nationwide could be accomplished with existing resources.

The study recognized the paucity of knowledge and understanding of the EMS workforce, attributing this lack of understanding to the nature and varied structure of EMS across the United States. It also recognized the unusually high incidence of occupational injuries among EMS providers.

The panel conducting the study faced many challenges, including defining a surveillance sys-

tem for EMS, gathering adequate data for analysis, identifying common themes among the literature for EMS injury patterns, reaching a consensus for a surveillance system, and developing a conceptual model for illness and injury surveillance for EMS.

From this study, it was concluded that no single data system exists that would be sufficient to meet this goal. However, many existing systems do contribute greatly at present and should be integrated to provide the necessary aggregate data. It was also recommended that this data should be shared with providers to improve outcomes. A national injury and illness surveillance program for EMS should be developed.

This effort exemplifies the importance of feasibility studies. More information on this study can be found on the NHTSA website.

CHAPTER REVIEW

Summary

Feasibility analysis is yet another useful process in the overall analytical approach in EMS. It differs from other analytical components in that its focus is on whether or not to proceed with an initiative or venture based on an organizational assessment with emphasis on economics, technical capabilities, legal compliance, and operational capacity. Although feasibility analysis has close ties to financial and cost-benefit analyses, it provides a somewhat different organizational perspective by examining qualitative factors and strategic planning goals.

Many less complex initiatives may be evaluated without a feasibility analysis or a reduced form of feasibility analysis, but any major decision or initiative should include a feasibility analysis given its unique nature. In the end, all analytical components should inform the final decision with appropriate weight of consideration.

WHAT WOULD YOU DO? Reflection

Having the crews and the management team behind this initiative removes much of the obstacles to its implementation. However, determining whether or not you have the financial and operational resources to support it and whether or not your customers will embrace it still remain unanswered questions. After conducting an economic feasibility analysis, you discover ample liquidity in the organization to support this initiative. The legal feasibility is promising, and the technical feasibility demands little supplemental support. The operational feasibility clearly demonstrates management and personnel support, and the initiative strongly supports the organization's mission and goals.

The feasibility analysis was most valuable by informing you of the potential threat that other organizations are contemplating the same initiative. Now it becomes a matter of time. With your resources aligned and the educational process underway, your organization will likely be the first to initiate this endeavor in your region. Delaying any longer would eliminate you from your strategic position.

Review Questions

1. Is it preferred that feasibility analysis be conducted solely or in conjunction with other analyses?
2. In what manner is feasibility analysis unique from other forms of analysis?
3. What are examples of intangible assets within a company that has value?
4. What does economic feasibility typically consist of?
5. What would be an example of an organization not having technical feasibility to pursue an endeavor?
6. How does concept testing differ from receptivity testing?
7. What is the scope of operations?
8. What is the internal environment of an organization, and how does it apply to a SWOT analysis?

9. How does SWOT analysis relate to the organization's goals and mission?

10. How can SWOT analysis help in better positioning an organization in the marketplace?

References

Harrison, J. P. (2010). *Essentials of Strategic Planning in Healthcare.* Chicago: Health Administration Press.

Shaw, P. L., and C. Elliott. (2012). *Quality and Performance Improvement in Healthcare,* 5th ed. Chicago: American Health Information Management Association.

Spath, P. (2009). *Introduction to Healthcare Quality Management.* Chicago: Health Administration Press.

Key Terms

concept testing The cognitive evaluation of an idea or initiative to forecast its viability; no actual product or service is delivered, but the conceptual content of the pursuit is examined.

cost-benefit analysis An assessment of a venture or initiative that determines its overall benefits versus its costs; includes a decision point as to whether or not to proceed; different from cost-effectiveness in that it considers societal values and must monetize all benefits and costs.

costs The value assigned to a service or product; in economics, a metric used to determine value in a decision-making process.

economic feasibility An analytical process as a component of feasibility analysis that determines financial prudence of a pursuit; often consists of financial analysis and cost-benefit analysis.

external environment The conditions outside of an organization; particularly the opportunities and threats that present to the organization.

feasibility study Identical to feasibility analysis, the analytical process designed to assist in deciding whether or not to proceed with a new initiative or venture based on its cost and value to the organization as well as the market's receptivity.

financial analysis An assessment of an organization's financial performance using financial statements, financial ratios, and interpretations of financial data.

force field analysis An extension of the SWOT analysis that attempts to disclose the driving forces behind the potential successes and hindrances that an organization may face.

gap analysis A comparative analysis of the organization's strengths and weakness against the profession's standards, the organization's goals, and the opportunities and threats that currently exist.

intangible A valued entity that has no physical form and cannot be easily measured, especially in monetary terms.

internal environment The conditions within the organization; particularly its strengths and weaknesses.

legal feasibility An analytical process as a component of feasibility analysis that explores the legal guidelines and regulatory restrictions that apply to the implementation of an initiative or venture.

operational feasibility An analytical process as a component of feasibility analysis that examines the organization's capacity and structure to determine congruence with a new initiative or venture; often includes strategic elements such as scope of operations, resource sufficiency, and SWOT analysis.

receptivity testing Similar to concept testing in feasibility analysis, except an actual prototype product or limited service to a subpopulation of the targeted clientele is tested for its utility and acceptability.

resource sufficiency Adequacy of assets of an organization, not only in financial terms, but also in access and availability of application.

scope of operations The capacity and breadth of an organization's operations in accordance with delivery models and practice standards.

SWOT analysis A component of operational feasibility that has its basis in strategic planning of an organization; it reveals the alignment potential of a new initiative or venture with the organization's mission, vision, and goals.

technical feasibility An analytical process as a component of feasibility analysis that assesses the functional ability of an organization to proceed with an initiative or venture; it examines the scope of performance and the organization's skill sets as applicable to the pursuit.

value Not just the monetary equivalency of a product or service, but also the quality it brings to the organization.

Writing the Final Report

8 CHAPTER

Objectives

After reading this chapter, the student should be able to:

8.1 Demonstrate an understanding of the importance of the final report on the overall analytical approach, what it represents, and what impact it may have on the decision maker.

8.2 Describe several approaches to writing the final report, and identify the most common format.

8.3 Identify the common sections in the final report, define their content, and explain the importance of their proper order.

8.4 Describe how the final section of the conclusion and recommendation should be crafted, specify what it should contain, and define its purpose.

Key Terms

breakeven analysis
cohort study
content analysis
cross-sectional study
dependent variables
financial ratios
financial statements
force field analysis
gap analysis
idiographic
impact analysis
  matrix

independent variables
key research question
logic model
longitudinal study
mind mapping
monetizations
multi-goal analysis
nomothetic
operationalization
prospective
  longitudinal study
qualitative analysis

quantitative analysis
resource sufficiency
  analysis
retrospective
  longitudinal study
scope of operations
  analysis
sensitivity analysis
SWOT analysis
units of analysis

The county commissioners have asked you, the lead administrator of your EMS agency, to investigate the opportunity to extend EMS coverage into the entire county as a single provider. You have spent months interviewing crew members, public officials, and local authorities. You have sent out surveys to the public and to the potential recipients of your service. You have conducted literature searches, examined your organization's financial statements, and conducted a cost-benefit analysis, an impact analysis, and a feasibility analysis on the proposed expansion. After all this time and effort, you now need to make a recommendation to the commissioners.

1. What is your best plan of action?
2. Should your recommendations be made in written format? If so, how should they appear?
3. What should be included and what should be omitted in your final report.
4. How should you proceed?

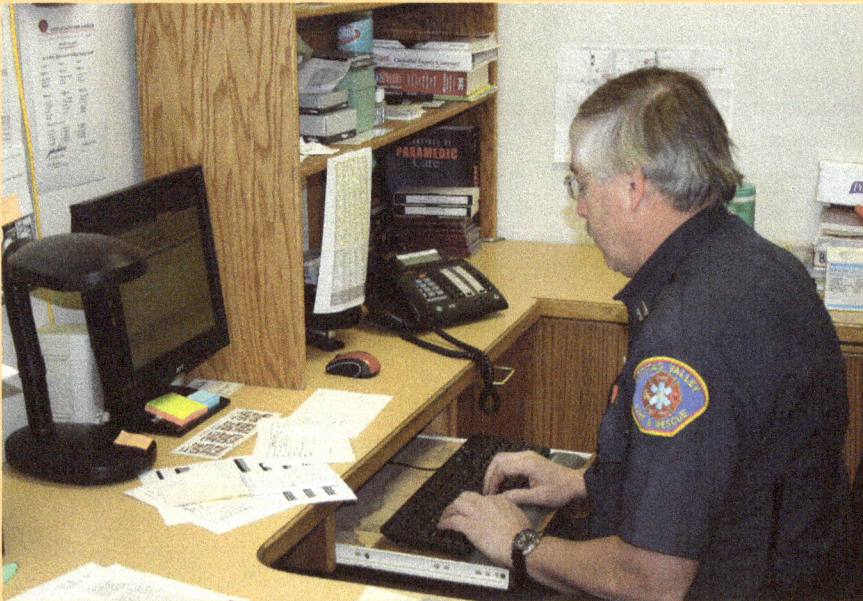

FIGURE 8.1 ■ Crafting the final report.

■ INTRODUCTION

Once all the analysis is complete, the results must be compiled into a single document that is reflective of all the analytical findings. This final step in the overall analytical process is essential as it communicates a summative conclusion of all the analytical components. In addition, it presents to the reader the convincing evidence acquired by the analyst and offers the final recommendation.

The final report is representative of all the time, effort, and individual systematic processes that underlie the analytical approach. It must be convincing, clear, well-supported, and unequivocal in its findings. The decision makers or stakeholders must be able to read the document, understand it, and arrive at the same conclusions and recommendations presented by the analyst. This document is so important that it is imperative for it to be done correctly. It would be counterproductive if an exhaustive analytical process revealed an effective solution alternative only for it to be ill represented in the final report, resulting in the correct alternative not being chosen. This chapter will describe the sections of the final report and how best to assemble them.

Side Bar

Final Report: Contents

A final report should look professional and assembled with careful thought. Often these formal reports are spiral bound; inserted into a labeled, three-ring binder; or enclosed in a plastic cover. Most reports should be assembled as follows:

* Title page containing the problem identification, date, and author of the report
* A table of contents listing the sections and associated page numbers
* A list of figures, if the report is large
* The contents of each section
* Any diagrams or charts embedded in the content
* A reference page, if necessary
* An appendix of any relevant information

Some final reports also provide an executive summary that summarizes the problem, the findings and a final recommendation. The report should follow the format as described in this chapter.

COMPILING THE FINAL REPORT—

There are many approaches to assembling all the information gathered through the analytical processes. One possible method is to simply construct summary reports of each of the analytical components to be assembled into a single document. If this approach is used, it is imperative that all the relevant data be recorded and that the conclusions drawn from that data be included. These individual analytical reports can then be rewritten into the final draft of the report using the approach described here.

Another method may be to document all the factual information without text or prose and insert that into the written content in a logical, progressive manner—once again following the approach described here. Whichever method you choose to assemble your findings, it is important that all the relevant data be included, that your report progresses logically from one concept or finding to the next, and that each component supports your final recommendation. It is acceptable if the analytical findings in some sections are not congruent with the findings in other sections, provided you can explain their variance. In the end, the final report should be convincing with a logical progression of thought.

SECTION ONE: IDENTIFICATION OF THE PROBLEM AND THE BACKGROUND

In this initial section of the final report, you present the nature of the problem to the readers. It is acceptable to initially report the perceived problem as long as the section describes the true nature of the problem. For example, it can be stated that the initial problem was perceived to be prolonged out-of-service times at the destination hospitals, but if the true nature of the problem was discovered to be lengthy delays in patient transfer of care to hospital staff, that should be stated as the true nature of the problem. This is important, for it is the true nature of the problem that will undergo the resultant analysis, not the perceived problem.

It is also important that the process employed to discern the true nature of the problem be described in this section. If **mind mapping** principles were utilized, they should be described and examples provided. If a **logic model** was constructed to illuminate the nature of the processes involved, it should be described and a representative logic model illustrated. Whatever means were used to reveal the true nature of the problem should be detailed in this section. Figure 8.2 depicts the logical order of this descriptive component.

If the perceived problem is the actual problem, the investigative process should still be described, but there is no need to focus on the discovery of the true nature since it remains the same. What is important is to ensure the reader that a systematic process was employed to investigate the problem to affirm its true nature. The format illustrated in Figure 8.2 should be followed even when the perceived and actual natures of the problem are identical.

This section is where any literature searches that were used to reveal the true nature of the problem can be included. It is important to note that this endeavor is not intended to resolve the problem. The literature searches are not conducted to discover a solution but, rather, the nature of the problem. Here, you can include summary information from the literature or even from subject interviews as to what the nature of the problem was believed to be. Similar accounts by other organizations or associations may be published in trade journals that will help in framing the nature of the problem. This is supportive information that should be included in this initial section. The interviews should be limited to only what the nature of the problem is believed to be and should not be intended for discovery of contributing or causal factors.

The nature of the problem should have some foundational description as well. Some background should be provided to help the reader understand why the problem became an issue and received so much attention. It is not expected (nor appropriate) that an attempt will be made to disclose the causation of the problem but, simply, to provide some background information. The causal factors will be revealed in the analysis later in the report.

The background is descriptive and often revealed in chronological fashion. That is, the suspected events or details that helped to initially create the perception of the problem

Problem Identification and Background	**Perceived Problem**—what the problem was believed to be initially
	Problem Identification Methods—how the true nature of the problem was discerned • Mind mapping • Logic models • Literature searches
	The True Nature of the Problem—what the actual problem was determined to be
	Background—some details of how the problem came to be; what events led to the realization of the problem

FIGURE 8.2 ■ Describing the identification of the problem.

should be described first and the remaining events or details described thereafter. Questions such as "How did this come to our attention?" and "Which event came first in our realization of this problem?" and "How long has this problem been plaguing us?" should be answered in the background of this section.

SECTION TWO: APPLYING THE PRINCIPLES OF RESEARCH

In this section, developing the analytical process will begin based on the true nature of the problem and application of the principles of research. This typically begins with translating the problem into a **key research question**. As always, the key research question, if answered, should lead to a resolution of the problem or an effective approach to an opportunity or venture. Most often a single research question should suffice. However, on occasion, it might be necessary to expand the question by posing some subordinate, secondary research questions. The secondary research questions should be closely related to and clarify the key research question.

From here, the methodology behind the research should be described. Begin with a general description of the type of research that was conducted, such as a **cross-sectional study**, a **qualitative analysis** or a **quantitative analysis**, and what time dimension was applied. For example, you may describe a retrospective **longitudinal study** that was conducted over 6 months or a prospective longitudinal **cohort study** that examined a group of paramedics over a period of 3 months. For the purposes of discovering a solution to a problem within an EMS context, it is most likely that the study will either be a cross-sectional study or a **retrospective longitudinal study**. A **prospective longitudinal study** takes time and money to effectively execute; by the very nature of the motivation for such an analysis, time is likely to be a valuable

commodity and so limited that it would not allow for a prospective investigation.

Although not essential, you may want to propose the theoretical approach that grounds your research analysis. You may frame the study in an **idiographic** or **nomothetic** manner, and you may indicate your approach as either inductive or deductive. In addition, any theory in which your research is grounded should be mentioned as well. Although essential in empirical analysis, these components may be somewhat relaxed in this application of research principles since they have purpose for the researcher and not for the decision maker or stakeholder.

In this methodology section, be sure to describe each of the variables and identify the **dependent variables** and **independent variables** accordingly. For each variable, detail the **operationalization** and the **units of analysis**. A simple description of the process is all that is necessary, but having some level of detail (e.g., what exactly the units of analysis were) is important.

The next logical step is to describe the data collection process. Provide explanation about what data collection methods were employed to satisfy the operationalization of the select variables. Provide your rationale for each collection method and the intended goals. In addition, give explanation about the number and nature of the targeted subjects. For example, you may write, "Fifty practicing paramedics in the state were surveyed by email to collect the necessary information." The intent here is to provide the reader with a clear understanding of who was selected to participate in the study, the number of subjects, what manner of data collection was employed, and some time line of collection.

It is also important to provide a sample of any data collection instrument that was used. If data were collected by means of an online or mailed survey, then the form should be included in the final report as an appendix and referenced in this section of the report. The same applies for any forms used for data extraction from documents or scripts used in the interview process.

Data collection methods are usually followed by the information results. This would include a compiled summary of all the variable results, often in a table format or simply a numerical synopsis. Providing the reader with the raw data helps to illustrate the nature, complexity, and magnitude of the endeavor and adds credibility to the conclusions. Just examining the data in this form can provide the reader with a general impression of the likely results.

If the research component of analysis involved a qualitative approach, then the results of the case study or **content analysis** should be included in this section. Providing the reader with a summary of the qualitative results helps to substantiate the conclusions drawn from the study and provides an unburdened synopsis of the content.

Following the results summary, provide interpretation of those results. Describe what the results mean and how you arrived at your conclusions. Often the interpretation is somewhat obvious and may involve a simple conclusion, but it is completely acceptable to provide some level of extrapolation of meaning and insightful interpretation of the results. For example, if the results demonstrated that the paramedic subjects in the study applied capnography and documented auscultatory findings following endotracheal intubation in all the cases, then it can be reasonably interpreted that their confirmation of tube placement was most likely accurate.

From the interpretation of data come conclusions that can be reasonably drawn from the information acquired. This entails taking the interpretations of all the findings and synthesizing general conclusions from them collectively. To do so may necessitate some explanation and rationale, but those

should be logical and clear in their development. Drawing conclusions from the research data has significant meaning to the overall analytical approach since it forms the foundation for all subsequent analytical processes that you may employ. If you intend to conduct a subsequent financial analysis, cost-benefit analysis, or impact analysis on the identified problem or initiative, then your research findings and conclusions should support that approach.

This section of the final report should also contain some explanation of the recognized or suspected threats to internal and external validity as well as any limitations of the study. Providing information related to any weaknesses of the study will help demonstrate credibility in the findings and illustrate the conscientious nature of the analysis.

Inclusion of the research component of your analysis in your final report follows a format similar to the problem identification and background approach. A summary of that format is illustrated in Figure 8.3. The elements are listed in their preferred order of inclusion in the report.

SECTION THREE: FINANCIAL ANALYSIS

If the nature of the problem or initiative demands a financial analysis, then those findings should be included in the next section of the final report. Most efforts to seek problem resolution or to decide on the best approach for an opportunity or initiative have an inherent financial concern. Therefore, this component merits some emphasis and should most likely follow any research component that was conducted.

Although the bulk of information in the financial analysis is derived from the **financial statements**, there is little reason to include the financial statements in the final report. They can be referenced, but the analysis findings, interpretations, and conclusions are all that

Research Component of Analysis	**Key Research Question**—a translation of the actual problem into questions that, when answered, provide a solution to the problem. This could also include secondary research questions.
	Research Methodology—how the research was conducted. It should include: • The type of research (quantitative, qualitative, or mixed methods) • The form of research (longitudinal prospective, longitudinal retrospective, cross-sectional, cohort, panel, etc.) • Theoretical approach (idiographic, nomothetic, inductive or deductive, etc.) • Variables (independent, dependent) • Methods of operationalization • Units of analysis • Data collection process (including collection instruments and methods)
	Results of Findings—what the data revealed in raw form
	Interpretation of Results—what the results mean, including synthesis of interpretation
	Threats to Validity and Limitations—what potential threats to internal and external validity exist and what limitations are recognized in the study
	Conclusions Drawn—compiling the interpretations into general conclusions from the research process

FIGURE 8.3   Describing the research components.

need to be reported in this final document. In select circumstances, it may be necessary to append the financial statements to the final report for reference. This may be particularly important for report readers who are financial decision makers. However, the financial analysis and interpretation always should be provided to the reader. Do not rely on the reader to make inferences from the financial statements.

The way your financial analysis is presented in the final document can vary in design, but it would likely include a summary interpretation of financial statement findings, presentation of **financial ratios**, and discussion of a **breakeven analysis**. Some additional information on pro forma statements may be necessary, and any reports on asset depreciation and assessments on time value of money (such as net present or future values) should be included, if appropriate.

Given the purpose behind financial analysis in decision making for problems or opportunities, it is probable that some report of liquidity, current assets, and debt-to-equity ratios would be essential. Profitability ratios, return on services, and interest coverage may also be beneficial. Figure 8.4 depicts the usual components of financial analysis in the final report.

SECTION FOUR: COST-BENEFIT ANALYSIS

In addition to financial analysis, a cost-benefit analysis is also a common component in the analytical approach to a problem or decision for an opportunity. Cost-benefit analysis contributes greatly toward the decision process by valuing options and weighing alternatives. If it is part of the overall analysis, it should be included in the final report following the financial analysis since the information provided by cost-benefit analysis is largely derived from the financial analysis component.

A cost-benefit analysis, as part of the overall analysis, should begin with a description of the process and the objectives of the

Financial Analysis Component	**Summary of Financial Statements**—a general description of findings from the financial statements with emphasis on elements that may impact decision making
	Financial Ratios—description of relevant financial ratios that inform the reader of financial statuses and potential risks. Some useful ratios include: • Current ratio and/or quick ratio • Asset turnover ratio and accounts receivable outstanding • Return on assets, return on services, and gross margin • Debt ratios and interest coverage
	Break-even Analysis—an interpretation of the point of profit versus cost in services delivered
	Summary of Pro Forma Statements—brief description of projected revenues, costs, and financial performances in the future
	Time Value of Money Assessments—descriptions of any determinations of asset depreciation, net present value of capital goods, or future value of capital goods

FIGURE 8.4 ■ Describing the financial analysis components.

analysis. The type of cost-benefit analysis should be described (*ex ante, ex post,* or *in media res*) as well as the methods employed.

When reporting the cost-benefit analysis in the final report, the content should be brief and concise. Inclusion of all the steps to cost-benefit analysis is unnecessary, and those that are included should only contain the essential elements that disclose the products of each step. Examples of what should be included are which alternatives are specified, which impacts are chosen, and what their **monetizations** are, any discounting to present value that was necessary,

and the results of a **sensitivity analysis**. Again, the purpose of the report is to summarize the results in an abbreviated fashion and not to describe the entire process.

For these abbreviated purposes, a cost-benefit analysis summary may consist of a compilation of all known benefits and their monetization values contrasted with the costs of each alternative. If discounting was necessary, that should be noted in the context. Ultimately, a recommendation should be made based on the findings of the cost-benefit analysis alone. Figure 8.5 illustrates the summary

Cost-Benefit Analysis Component	**Type of Cost-Benefit Analysis**—describe the type of CBA conducted
	Elements of the Cost-Benefit Analysis—a brief summary of the results of each step of the CBA that is necessary. It *may* include: • Alternatives selected • List of benefits and costs to be included • Description of the measurement indicators/impacts • Summary of the monetization of each impact for each alternative • Description of any discounting or net present value determinations • Results of any sensitivity analyses conducted
	Recommendation—the recommendation based upon the cost-benefit analysis *only*

FIGURE 8.5 ■ Describing the cost-benefit analysis components.

steps to the cost-benefit analysis in the final report.

SECTION FIVE: IMPACT ANALYSIS

In some instances, determining the impacts from various alternatives and their consequences may prove to be very useful in an overall analysis. Therefore, impact analysis may become part of the final report. If so, its position is most logical following the cost-benefit analysis since many of the concepts of impact analysis have parallel origins to cost-benefit analysis and many of the measures are the same.

Once again, all that needs to be reported are the summary findings and not a detailed description of the processes involved. The foundational basis of the impact analysis should be described and the approach chosen (almost always a **multi-goal analysis**) discussed. With that, the specific primary goals of the solution or opportunity should be defined and each alternative specified in this component of the final report.

Once you have described the goals, identify the impact categories and how they will be valued. The primary goals, alternative solutions, impact categories, and resultant values of each should be clearly communicated and apparent in comparisons. A summary table or an **impact analysis matrix** will often serve these purposes well. If an impact analysis matrix is included in the final report, some descriptive explanation of the categories, columns, and rows would be necessary.

From this, a discussion of the evaluative processes of the outcomes should be presented. A recommendation should be offered from the impact analysis only. As you progress through the final report, each section should have its own conclusion, and all conclusions should be drawn together in the final summary and recommendation of the report. Figure 8.6 illustrates the components of the impact analysis section of the final report.

SECTION SIX: FEASIBILITY ANALYSIS

In this last section before the conclusion and recommendation, the findings from the feasibility analysis (if conducted) should be presented. When a decision between several options is necessary, a feasibility analysis often proves to be quite useful.

This section should begin with the type of feasibility analysis that was conducted. If a

Impact Analysis Component	
	Summary Description of the Impact Analysis—describe the type of impact analysis conducted and why it was deemed necessary
	Describe the Elements of the Impact Analysis and Generate an Impact Analysis Matrix—provide a brief description of the components of the impact analysis and a summary of the results. If an impact analysis matrix is included, make reference to it and explain the findings. This *should* include: • Primary goals of the solution/initiative • Alternative options • Impact categories • Description of the valuation methods of each impact category • Summary results of each impact value for each alternative solution
	Interpretation and Recommendation—the summary interpretation of the impact analysis and a resultant recommendation based upon the impact analysis *only*

FIGURE 8.6 ■ Describing the impact analysis components.

financial analysis or a cost-benefit analysis was already completed, then an economic feasibility analysis is unnecessary. There may be a need to report on a technical feasibility analysis or even a legal feasibility analysis. However, it is almost always important to include an operational feasibility analysis with emphasis on its inherent components.

Once again, the report should include only the summary results of each type of feasibility analysis. The technical feasibility analysis may report on the results of any concept or receptivity testing and the legal feasibility on any official determinations as to permissibility and regulatory compliance issues. The operational feasibility report should include the results of each subcomponent: the **scope of operations analysis**, the **resource sufficiency analysis**, the **SWOT analysis** (an analysis of Strengths, Weaknesses, Opportunities, and Threats), and any other subordinate analyses (such as **force field analysis** or **gap analysis**). It may also be useful to include a SWOT analysis matrix or a force field analysis chart in the appendix of the report. Figure 8.7 demonstrates the descriptive components of the feasibility analyses in the final report.

SECTION SEVEN: CONCLUSION AND RECOMMENDATION

In this final step of the written report, a recommendation should be made to the reader and, likely, the decision maker. The recommendation is a formulation of multiple interpretations and conclusions drawn from the many aspects of the overall analytical approach. This recommendation begins with a true understanding of the problem with a resultant empirically sound investigation into the causal and mitigating factors that either created or influenced its existence. A thorough financial analysis and cost-benefit analysis were likely conducted to illustrate the benefits of a new opportunity or the costs of a problem resolution. In any given analytical approach, an impact analysis and a feasibility analysis may have been conducted on alternative solutions to the problem or opportunities facing the organization. Whatever the extent of analysis, at least several viable alternatives were created through this process.

Now, the task at hand is to make the final recommendation. This task is made simpler and more reliable by the overall analytical approach based on multiple analytical processes. With

Feasibility Analysis Component	**Type and Rationale Behind the Feasibility Analysis**—describe the types of feasibility analyses conducted and why they were deemed necessary
	Describe the Elements of the Feasibility Analyses—provide a brief description of each of the types of feasibility analysis conducted and a summary of the results. This *may* include: • Economic feasibility analysis (if no financial and cost-benefit analyses were conducted) • Technical feasibility analysis • Legal feasibility analysis • Operational feasibility analysis, including scope of operations, resource sufficiency, SWOT analysis, and any other subordinate analyses
	Interpretation and Recommendation—the summary interpretation of the feasibility analyses and a resultant recommendation based upon the feasibility analyses *only*

FIGURE 8.7 ■ Describing the feasibility analyses components.

each analytical component, a solution or several solutions will become apparent. Now, it is a matter of the analyst taking the conclusion of each component that was previously analyzed and compiling those findings into a single recommendation for a solution. In many cases of comprehensive analysis, the concluding solution is often the most prevalent solution for each of the analytical components. In some analyses, it is a matter of reconciliation of the best solutions.

Whatever the choice becomes, it is based on the real data that each analytical approach utilized and is a product of the multiple inputs into the solution. The final recommendation should be derived logically and with appropriate emphasis on the most important analyses. It should also take into consideration the political impact of each alternative solution and the preferences of the client or stakeholder. An illustration of the overall process is demonstrated in Figure 8.8.

Problem Identification and Background	**Perceived Problem**—what the problem was believed to be initially
	Problem Identification Methods—how the true nature of the problem was discerned. • Mind mapping • Logic models • Literature searches
	The True Nature of the Problem—what the actual problem was determined to be
	Background—some details of how the problem came to be; what events led to the realization of the problem
Research Component of Analysis	**Key Research Question**—a translation of the actual problem into questions that, when answered, provide a solution to the problem. This could also include secondary research questions.
	Research Methodology—how the research was conducted. It should include: • The type of research (quantitative, qualitative, or mixed methods) • The form of research (longitudinal prospective, longitudinal retrospective, cross-sectional, cohort, panel, etc.) • Theoretical approach (idiographic, nomothetic, inductive, or deductive, etc.) • Variables (independent, dependent) • Methods of operationalization • Units of analysis • Data collection process (including collection instruments and methods)
	Results of Findings—what the data revealed in raw form
	Interpretation of Results—what the results mean, including synthesis of interpretation
	Threats to Validity and Limitations—what potential threats to internal and external validity exist and what limitations are recognized in the study
	Conclusions Drawn—compilation of the interpretations from the research process into general conclusions

FIGURE 8.8 ■ Summary description of the analyses components.

Financial Analysis Component	**Summary of Financial Statements**—a general description of findings from the financial statements with emphasis on elements that may impact decision making
	Financial Ratios—description of relevant financial ratios that inform the reader of financial statuses and potential risks. Some useful ratios include: • Current ratio and/or quick ratio • Asset turnover ratio and accounts receivable outstanding • Return on assets, return of services, and gross margin • Debt ratios and interest coverage
	Breakeven Analysis—an interpretation of the point of profit versus cost in services delivered
	Summary of Pro Forma Statements—brief description of projected revenues, costs, and financial performances in the future
	Time Value of Money Assessments—descriptions of any determinations of asset depreciation, net present value of capital goods, or future value of capital goods
Cost-Benefit Analysis Component	**Type of Cost-Benefit Analysis**—describe the type of CBA conducted
	Elements of the Cost-Benefit Analysis—a brief summary of the results of each step of the CBA that is necessary. It *may* include: • Alternatives selected • List of benefits and costs to be included • Description of the measurement indicators/impacts • Summary of the monetization of each impact for each alternative • Description of any discounting or net present value determinations • Results of any sensitivity analyses conducted
	Recommendation—the recommendation based upon the cost-benefit analysis *only*
Impact Analysis Component	**Summary Description of the Impact Analysis**—describe the type of impact analysis conducted and why it was deemed necessary
	Describe the Elements of the Impact Analysis and Generate an Impact Analysis Matrix—provide a brief description of the components of the impact analysis and a summary of the results. If an impact analysis matrix is included, make reference to it and explain the findings. This *should* include: • Primary goals of the solution/initiative • Alternative options • Impact categories • Description of the valuation methods of each impact category • Summary results of each impact value for each alternative solution
	Interpretation and Recommendation—the summary interpretation of the impact analysis and a resultant recommendation based upon the impact analysis *only*

FIGURE 8.8 ■ (*Continued*)

Feasibility Analysis Component	**Type and Rationale Behind the Feasibility Analysis**—describe the types of feasibility analyses conducted and why they were deemed necessary
	Describe the Elements of the Feasibility Analyses—provide a brief description of each of the types of feasibility analyses conducted and a summary of the results. This *may* include: • Economic feasibility analysis (if no financial and cost-benefit analyses were conducted) • Technical feasibility analysis • Legal feasibility analysis • Operational feasibility analysis, including scope of operations, resource sufficiency, SWOT analysis, and any other subordinate analyses
	Interpretation and Recommendation—the summary interpretation of the feasibility analyses and a resultant recommendation based upon the feasibility analyses *only*
Conclusion and Final Recommendation	

FIGURE 8.8 ■ (*Continued*)

CHAPTER REVIEW

Summary

The final report is a summation of all the efforts and results from each component of the overall analytical approach. It provides the reader and decision maker with substantive information that is cogent, concise, and logical, leading to a reliable recommendation. When properly prepared, the reader is not burdened with the details of the inherent processes but, instead, has the opportunity to appreciate the summary of the analyses. In this way, the decision maker can support the recommendation with comfort and confidence, for it is likely that the best solution to the problem or the best alternative approach to the opportunity has been chosen.

WHAT WOULD YOU DO? Reflection

After careful contemplation, you begin crafting your final document. You realize that such an important decision with so much information must be presented in a written report. You decide to follow the logical progression of processes that you employed in your overall analytical approach. In doing so, you summarize your findings for each analytical component and then document that summary in a logical and fluid progression of thoughts.

With each component, you reveal the recommendation of that analytical process and, in the end, they all point to one conclusion and recommendation: to proceed with the expansion. Your analysis not only revealed the plausibility of the expansion but also the projected costs and the probable benefits. You feel confident that the county commissioners will not only accept your recommendation but will feel confident that it is the best decision.

Review Questions

1. What goals should the final report expect to accomplish?
2. What should one do if an analytical process results in a conclusion that does not support all other conclusions and the final recommendation?
3. If the true nature of the problem turns out to be completely different from the initially perceived problem, should the initial problem even be reported?
4. What role do literature searches have in the final report?
5. If a financial analysis and a cost-benefit analysis have been conducted as part of an overall analytical approach, is it necessary to conduct a financial feasibility study?
6. When reporting on the research principles employed in the investigative analysis, when should the type of research study be described?
7. What value does describing the theoretical nature of the research have to the reader or decision maker in the final report?
8. If data collection occurred as a result of focus group interviews and online surveys, how should this information be portrayed in the final report?
9. How should the impact analysis be reported in the final report document?
10. Of the various forms of feasibility analyses, which is likely to be of greatest value in the final report?

References

Alred, G. J., C. T. Brusaw, and W. E. Oliu. (2012). *Handbook of Technical Writing,* 10th ed. Boston: Bedford/St. Martin's.

Blake, G., and R. W. Bly. (1992). *The Elements of Business Writing: A Guide to Writing Clear, Concise Letters, Memos, Reports, Proposals, and Other Business Documents.* Essex, UK: Longman Press.

Kupsh, J., and R. Rhodes. (2010). *Report Writing: A Survival Guide,* Bloomington, IN: Xlibris Corporation.

Mort, S. (1995). *Professional Report Writing.* Farnham, UK: Gower Publishing, Ltd..

Riordan, D. G. (2014). *Technical Report Writing Today.* Independence, KY: Wadsworth Cengage Learning.

Van Laan, K., and J. T. Hackos. (2012). *The Insider's Guide to Technical Writing.* Laguna Hills, CA: XML Press.

Key Terms

breakeven analysis An analytical process that determines at what point the revenue of services covers all the costs of operations (fixed and variable costs).

cohort study A longitudinal study whereby the study group has some commonality or bond characteristic among the subjects.

content analysis An analytical process for the written word whereby concepts or repeating themes are identified and coded for later analysis.

cross-sectional study A type of investigational study that examines data at one moment in time; it represents a "snapshot" of the events in time.

dependent variable The central variable of interest in the study; the variable that answers the key research question; the variable that is *dependent* on the other, independent variables to exist or vary in value.

financial ratios An analytical tool in financial analysis that compares elements of the financial statements through proportions and relationships.

financial statements Documents in an organization that detail financial data; includes the balance sheet, the income statement, and the cash flow statement.

force field analysis An extension of the SWOT analysis that attempts to disclose the driving forces behind the potential successes and hindrances that an organization may face.

gap analysis A comparative analysis of the organization's strengths and weakness against the profession's standards, the organization's goals, and the opportunities and threats that currently exist.

idiographic An investigative study approach to explanation whereby an exhaustive assessment of all the possible causes of an event or phenomenon is conducted.

impact analysis matrix A summary table of the primary goals, alternative solutions, and impacts of each for purposes of outcome comparison.

independent variables Variables in a study that are presumed to cause or alter the value of the dependent variable(s); variables of interest that are the subject of data collection in a study.

key research question The guiding interrogative principle behind the study; the problem for which a solution is being sought in a general question format.

logic model A conceptual illustration that demonstrates the elemental components to a complex process to render a relational understanding and an association among those components.

longitudinal study An investigative study that examines data over a period of time to determine changes over time.

mind mapping A conceptual application that illustrates relationships and associations to various elements within a common theme. The process includes a colorful depiction of components and a branching hierarchy of ideas and concepts.

monetization A process of valuing an impact through the metric of money.

multi-goal analysis A type of impact analysis that examines alternatives through the lens of primary goals; one of the more popular and effective methods of impact analysis.

nomothetic An investigative study approach to explanation whereby the most influential factors are examined closely, using

probabilities and similar analyses for explanation.

operationalization The method or process to be employed in measuring the values of the variables of interest; to make the variable contributory in the study.

prospective longitudinal study An investigative study that examines data over time in the future.

qualitative analysis A fundamental research design that studies events or phenomenon of a non-numerical nature, typically of a behavioral or communication nature, and attempts to disclose underlying meanings and patterns of relationships.

quantitative analysis A fundamental research design that studies events or phenomena of a numerical nature, typically through observations, interventions, precise measurements, and statistical probability predictions, to disclose underlying relationships of causality.

resource sufficiency analysis An assessment of an organization intended to determine the adequacy of assets of an organization, not only in financial terms but also in access and availability of application.

retrospective longitudinal study An investigative study that examines data over time in a retrospective manner; often derived through the examination of documents and records.

scope of operations analysis An assessment of an organization intended to determine the capacity and breadth of an organization's operations in accordance with delivery models and practice standards.

sensitivity analysis A step in cost-benefit analysis that attempts to measure the consequences of the impact categories of various alternatives and the effect each has on the others by acknowledging the presence of uncertainty.

SWOT analysis Strengths, Weaknesses, Opportunities, and Threats; a component of operational feasibility that has its basis in strategic planning of an organization; it reveals the alignment potential of a new initiative or venture with the organization's mission, vision, and goals.

units of analysis An important element in study design that specifies the "what" or "whom" that is being studied.

Glossary

accelerated depreciation A method of asset depreciation that places larger portions of depreciation in the early years of the expected life of the item either for accounting or tax deduction purposes.

accounts payable Appears on the balance sheet and represents obligations the organization has to creditors and suppliers.

accrued expenses Expenses that have come to term or have been already incurred; a sum of all the current expenses.

accumulated depreciation Appears on the balance sheet as the total depreciation of all assets for the period under review.

activities The second level of a logic model that associates processes of inputs to achieve outputs.

agency theory The environmental setting or institutional framework in which the problem resides and in which the analysis and decision making will be conducted.

analytical design The basic structure of the analytical approach, based on general principles of research. The analytical design is variable and dependent on circumstances and informational needs.

assets On the balance sheet, assets are tangible items that have associated value; often of property, buildings, and equipment.

asset turnover ratio A financial ratio that demonstrates the effectiveness at which assets in the organization can generate service revenue.

attrition effects A form of internal validity threat whereby subject withdraw or fall-out from the study occurs before the study ends, causing erroneous outcomes.

balance sheet One of the more commonly utilized financial statements; it reveals the values of the assets, liabilities, and shareholder's equity at a given point in time.

bounded rationality The limitations of human thought that prevents full resolution of problems due to their complexity, the incomplete nature of information, the natural differences among people's preferences and beliefs, and the conflicts of value held by many people.

breakeven analysis An analytical process that determines at what point the revenue of services covers all the costs of operations (fixed and variable costs).

breakeven point In breakeven analysis, the exact point where revenue or retained earnings meet the total costs of operation; where there is no profit and no losses.

capital stock The investment into a business for start-up and add-on growth by owners of the company.

cash disbursements Found on the cash flow statement, payments made to vendors that lower the cash asset and the accounts payable sections of the balance sheet.

cash flow statement A financial statement that tracks the movement of cash through an organization over a period of time; focuses on operations, investments, and financing.

cash receipts Also referred to as collections, the item on the cash flow statement that reveals the cash received from doing business.

causality Creating an effect; being responsible for changing or creating a variable; a foundational component of statistical analysis.

coding A process of recording or denoting a value in the qualitative assessment of a document or transcription; transferring raw data into standardized forms for analysis.

cohort study A longitudinal study whereby the study group has some commonality or bond characteristic among the subjects.

concept testing The cognitive evaluation of an idea or initiative to forecast its viability; no actual product or service is delivered, but the conceptual content of the pursuit is examined.

concurrent research Research that is conducted at the same time as other research or during research design development; if qualitative and quantitative research are being conducted simultaneously (mixed methods), they are concurrent (if conducted serially, they are sequential).

confirmation biases Making choices based on the influences of a personal agenda.

confounding effects When the value of one (typically unknown) independent variable affects the value of another independent variable; when an extraneous, unknown variable covaries with another variable of interest.

content analysis An analytical process for the written word whereby concepts or repeating themes are identified and coded for later analysis.

continuous variable A numerical variable that has the potential for progressive value change, such as age.

correlation When one variable influences another variable with change; a criterion for proper variable selection whereby the chosen (independent) variable influences the dependent variable when change comes about.

cost-benefit analysis An analytical process, financially based, that compares the aggregate net benefits of an endeavor with its aggregate net expenses; an assessment of a venture or initiative that determines its overall benefits versus its costs; includes a decision point as to whether or not to proceed; different from cost-effectiveness in that it considers societal values and must monetize all benefits and costs.

cost-effectiveness analysis Similar to cost-benefit analysis, this form of analysis does not consider societal impacts, particularly the value of human life; any analysis that fails to monetize impacts or consider human life impacts may qualify for cost-effectiveness analysis.

costs The value assigned to a service or product; in economics, a metric used to determine value in a decision-making process.

costs of services Typically costs of goods sold on the income statement in production companies; those costs and expenses associated with the production or delivery of services.

cross-sectional study A type of investigational study that examines data at one moment in time; it represents a "snapshot" of the events in time.

current assets Found on the balance sheet, the items of value that are expected to be turned into cash in the short term (usually less than 1 year).

current debt On the balance sheet under the liabilities column, the portion of debt that is due for collection in the short term (usually under 1 year).

current liabilities Found on the balance sheet, current liabilities are bills that are due in the short term (usually under 1 year) and typically consist of accounts payable, accrued expenses, current debt, and income taxes that are currently due for payment.

current ratio A common measure of an organization's liquidity that relates the sum of the current assets to the sum of the current liabilities.

data collection instrument Any device or construct that enables data collection; the most common forms are surveys, questionnaires, or tick forms.

debt ratio Also known as the debt-to-assets ratio, reveals an organization's outstanding debt obligations to total assets; used as a measure of financial leverage.

deductive approach A theoretical structure of inquiry whereby a general concept, belief, or theory is used to guide the research and detailed factors are analyzed to determine if they support the overall theory or belief; from the general to the particulars.

dependent variable The central variable of interest in the study; the variable that answers the key research question; the variable that is dependent on the other, independent variables to exist or vary in value.

discounting future value A means of applying the concept of time value of money whereby the present value of future money is determined.

double-declining balance depreciation A method of depreciation of goods whereby the depreciation rate of the good is doubled for the expected life of the asset; a means that places the greater depreciation in earlier years for an accelerated depreciation.

EBIT Earnings Before Interest and Taxes; a measure of money revenue that is conservative.

economic feasibility An analytical process as a component of feasibility analysis that determines financial prudence of a pursuit; often consists of financial analysis and cost-benefit analysis.

empirical process A process of formal analysis that abides by rules of structure and procedure to render valid and reliable data.

ending cash balance Found on the cash flow statement, it represents the final registration on the statement; the result of the beginning cash balance, plus any cash received, and minus any cash spent.

equity Found on the balance sheet, the recorded ownership claim of common and preferred stock for an organization's stakeholders.

evidence-based practice Conducting an activity that has reliable, empirical evidence to support its implementation.

ex ante cost-benefit analysis A cost-benefit analysis that is conducted before the project, problem resolution, opportunity endeavor, or event.

ex ante process In impact analysis, when the analytical process occurs before the problem is resolved, opportunity is begun, or a project is launched.

ex post cost-benefit analysis A cost-benefit analysis that is conducted after the project, problem resolution, opportunity endeavor, or event.

ex post process In impact analysis, when the analytical process occurs after the problem is resolved, opportunity is begun, or a project is launched as a means of evaluating success.

experimental design A form of quantitative research that allows randomization of subjects or interventions to study groups.

experimenter bias A threat to internal validity whereby the researcher (tester) conducting the data collection introduces selection bias into the study by behaving differently for some subjects or data elements than for others.

external environment The conditions outside of an organization; particularly the opportunities and threats that present to the organization

external validity Also known as generalization; having the quality of being able to apply the findings of the study from the select study population group to other, similar groups outside of the study; universal application of conclusions.

feasibility analysis An analytical process that helps to determine if an endeavor can be implemented given the nature of the organization, the mission of the organization, and the operational environment; often compared to a SWOT analysis.

feasibility study Identical to feasibility analysis, the analytical process designed to assist in deciding whether or not to proceed with a new initiative or venture based on its cost and value to the organization as well as the market's receptivity.

feedback loops Informational inputs into the processes of a logic model from resultant events. Feedback loops can occur anywhere in the logic model to inform an earlier process or activity.

financial analysis An assessment of an organization's financial performance using financial statements, financial ratios, and interpretations of financial data.

financial ratios An analytical tool in financial analysis that compares elements of the financial statements through proportions and relationships.

financial statements Documents in an organization that detail financial data; includes the balance sheet, the income statement, and the cash flow statement.

fixed asset purchases Found on the cash flow statement, the amount of money spent purchasing assets (property, buildings, and equipment).

fixed assets Found on the balance sheet, properties or items of value to the organization that are not intended for sale and usually used over and over again in the production of services (or sales).

fixed costs Any cost that doesn't vary in value or amount with changes in operations over time.

focus group interviews A form of qualitative inquiry that involves the researcher gathering interview data from groups of individuals simultaneously; typically, the individuals have some common link or association (e.g., members of a group, the general public, groups of co-workers, etc.).

force field analysis An extension of the SWOT analysis that attempts to disclose the driving forces behind the potential successes and hindrances that an organization may face.

future value The present-day value of a cost or benefit in the future with a known compound interest rate and period of time in years.

GAAP Generally Accepted Accounting Procedures; procedures, conventions, and practices that are established by the Financial Accounting Standards Board (FASB) for the preparation and reporting of financial statements.

gap analysis A comparative analysis of the organization's strengths and weakness against the profession's standards, the organization's goals, and the opportunities and threats that currently exist.

general and administrative expenses Found on the income statement, costs not directly associated with the delivery of services or operations; often a significant source of indirect expenses; includes administrative expenses, clerical, preparation, and day-to-day costs such as utilities.

gross margin Found on the income statement, it represents the amount of money left over from the revenue of services delivered minus the cost to deliver those services; also called gross profit.

gross profit Found on the income statement, it represents the amount of money left over from the revenue of services delivered minus the cost to deliver those services; also called gross margin.

hawthorne effect An alteration in the subjects' behavior secondary to knowing that they are being assessed or tested; discovered at a production plant Illinois (Hawthorne Plant) and described by Elton Mayo.

history effects Events or behavioral changes that occur to subjects throughout the duration of the study that may affect the outcome under study.

idiographic An investigative study approach to explanation whereby an exhaustive assessment of all the possible causes of an event or phenomenon is conducted.

impact analysis An analytical approach, adopted from policy analysis, that enables a systematic assessment of alternative solutions to a problem or opportunity on the basis of the varying goals and impact categories of each solution and how those choices will impact the organization, community, or society in general.

impact analysis matrix An illustrative table that details each of the primary goals and their associated impact categories against each of the problem solution alternatives; summarizing the impact analysis in a table format.

impact categories Ways that the primary goals can be measured; occurrences or events that result from the accomplishment of the primary goals.

impacts A consequence to an event or decision that can be either an input or output and can be categorized and measured.

incidental services Sometimes found on the income statement, representing services provided that are not directly linked to the mission of the organization, but may have value and even generate income.

income from operations The revenue generated by the activities purposed by the organization in its delivery of services; derived from the gross margin minus the operating expenses.

income statement One of the financial statements that provide information on the revenues and matching costs for an organization during a specific time period; a report of the income earned by the organization; sometimes referred to as an operating statement or profit and loss statement.

income taxes payable Part of the current liabilities on the balance sheet that indicates the current tax liabilities.

independent variable A variable in a study that is presumed to cause or alter the value of the dependent variable; variables of interest that are the subject of data collection in a study.

inductive approach A study approach whereby pieces of information are gathered through data collection into aggregate form to create a theory or central belief that offers explanation in the study; going from the particulars to the general.

informational asymmetry A circumstance whereby one party has more or better information than another party and uses that information to his advantage; often found when one entity has authority over another, as in the principal-agent relationship.

in media res cost-benefit analysis A cost-benefit analysis that is conducted during the project, problem resolution, opportunity endeavor, or event.

inputs A type of impact (asset or factor) that contributes to the development of the alternative or venture; the first level of a logic model that lists the resources and constituent components to the process.

institutional review board A committee at universities and colleges comprised of professionals who oversee studies on human subjects to protect their rights and enforce medical ethics.

intangible A valued entity that has no physical form and cannot be easily measured, especially in monetary terms.

integrated analytical report The final report of the analytical approach. It is concise, detailed, informative, and well referenced. Minimally, it consists of an introduction, background, problem identification, analytical design description, data collection methods, results and interpretations, alternative solutions, and recommendations.

interest coverage A financial analysis tool that reveals the relationship of periodic interest expense to operating income before or after taxes; often used to judge an organization's ability to pay interest on loans.

interest on income Earnings outside of operational income, often from interest on investments or cash dividends.

internal environment The conditions within the organization; particularly its strengths and weaknesses.

internal validity The quest of quantitative (and qualitative) research to ensure that the study design provides an explanation of causality between the independent and dependent variables.

kaldor-hicks criterion A condition of Pareto efficiency that states a decision, solution, project, or alternative should be chosen if the individuals benefiting from it are able to compensate those who are made worse off by it and still be better off.

key research question The guiding interrogative principle behind the study; the problem for which a solution is being sought in a general question format.

latent content In content analysis, discerning the underlying meaning for words or phrases intended by the interviewee; a subjective interpretation of the interviewee's meanings in statements.

legal feasibility An analytical process as a component of feasibility analysis that explores the legal guidelines and regulatory restrictions that apply to the implementation of an initiative or venture.

leverage The practice of using organizational resources (usually assets or equity) to achieve greater profits or revenue; a means of magnifying the profits from increases in the volume of services through fixed assets or equity; usually either operating leverage or financial leverage.

leverage ratios Financial analysis tools that measure how much of the company's assets are financed with debt to demonstrate an organization's "equity cushion" and how much the organization can tolerate additional debt.

liabilities A category on the balance sheet that illustrates the obligations the organization has to its creditors and vendors.

likert scale A scale format used in surveys and similar data collection instruments that provides the respondent with the option of indicating a valued response, typically on a numerical scale.

liquidity The ability to convert assets (current) to cash in the short term; also known as solvency.

liquidity ratios Financial analytical tools that demonstrate an organization's ability to convert current assets to cash in the short term.

literature searches Careful examinations of the current and past professionally published documents that can inform a situation or problem. These are often conducted through a professional search engine or database.

logic model A conceptual illustration that demonstrates the elemental components to a complex process to render a relational understanding and an association among those components.

long-term debt Any financial payment obligation that extends beyond 1 year.

long-term liabilities Expenses to an organization that extend beyond 1 year in duration; often found on the balance sheet.

longitudinal study An investigative study that examines data over a period of time to determine changes over time.

manifest content In content analysis, the obvious and declared meaning of statements from the interviewee taken for their face value, typically through a summation of occurrences in the interview.

maturation effects The consequences of when subjects in a study undergo natural changes that would occur otherwise in the study that may influence the study's outcome through threats of internal validity.

mind mapping A conceptual application that illustrates relationships and associations to various elements within a common theme. The process includes a colorful depiction of components and a branching hierarchy of ideas and concepts.

mixed methods design A research design that incorporates both quantitative as well as qualitative components; an approach that is becoming increasingly popular in its value and impact.

monetization Placing a money value on an impact (after it's been quantified).

monte carlo sensitivity analysis A form of sensitivity analysis that approximates impact values based on probabilities and also accounts for uncertainties by randomly altering impact values to determine statistically likely outcomes.

multi-goal analysis A type of impact analysis that examines alternatives by identifying the goals necessary for resolution and comparing the impacts that occur for each goal; one of the more popular and effective methods of impact analysis.

mutually exclusive In impact analysis, a condition of problem alternatives whereby each solution alternative is unique from the other and not a variation of one theme.

net benefits The value remaining after considering all of the benefits and deducting all of the costs.

net borrowings Found on the cash flow statement, it is the difference between any new borrowings in a time period and the amount already paid back.

net current assets The current assets of an organization less the current liabilities; also known as working capital.

net income The final registration on the income statement that reveals either a positive cash reserve or a negative cash loss; the difference between the combined income from operations (gross margin less operating expense) and interest income and the amount paid out in taxes.

net present value The difference between the present value of all of the benefits, less the present value of all of the costs; present value is determined by discounting the future value.

net sales (or net services) Found on the income statement, the amount of revenue earned in a period of time from sales (in a production company) or services delivered (in a service company).

net worth The recorded value of shareholder's equity on the balance sheet; same as shareholder's equity.

nomothetic explanation An investigative study approach to explanation whereby the most influential factors are examined closely, using probabilities and similar analyses for explanation.

non-cash transactions Financial exchange activities that do not involve cash flow; activities that may involve action, but do not immediately add to the cash on hand and will not appear on the cash flow statement.

nonspuriousness A criterion for variable selection that specifies that the variable of interest has no other outside factors of influence on the outcome variable; the relationship between the independent variable and dependent variable is uncorrupted.

operating expenses Found on the income statement, those expenditures that a company incurs in its operations to earn income; often includes service delivery, marketing, incidental services, and general and administrative expenses.

operating leverage The effect that changes in volume of services from operations has on profits caused by fixed costs; any change in operational practices that offers financial advantages.

operational feasibility An analytical process as a component of feasibility analysis that examines the organization's capacity and structure to determine congruence with a new initiative or venture; often includes strategic elements such as scope of operations, resource sufficiency, and SWOT analysis.

operationalization The method or process to be employed in measuring the values of the variables of interest; to make the variable contributory in the study.

outcomes The eventual result of the entire process in a logic model. Outcomes may be short term, intermediate term, or long term.

outputs A type of impact (asset or factor) that is produced as a result of an alternative or venture under consideration; the third level of a logic model that is the product of the activities applied to the inputs (or resources) in a process; often measureable and often short lived.

panel study A longitudinal study whereby the study group is followed over a period of time with a focus on some characteristic common to each of them; they may be disparate otherwise and not of a common group; similar to a cohort study.

pareto efficiency A form of efficiency in welfare microeconomics that requires that any alternative allocation in the distribution of a good or service which will make any individual better off will not make anyone else worse off.

political feasibility The acceptability of a proposed solution to stakeholders and decision makers regardless of its effectiveness to resolve the problem.

present value The value today of a future asset or sum of money calculated by discounting the future value to today's value.

primary goals The identified purposes to be accomplished by each alternative solution; what the resolution hopes to achieve.

pro forma statements Financial statements that project revenues and costs based on formulated conditions and trended expectations over a period of time.

problem identification The initial step in the analytical process; it ensures the correct identification of a problem or opportunity through a variety of analyses.

profitability ratios Financial analysis tools that relate profits to some other component of financial information; often referred to as "return on" ratios as they reveal the profit return on another financial aspect.

profit margin A financial performance measure derived by comparing the net services from the income statement with the net income; sometimes referred to as gross margin.

prospective longitudinal study An investigative study that examines data over time in the future.

prospective research A form of longitudinal research that looks to the future for data collection and results; these studies are very effective as the design is preliminarily determined and all controls can be put into place before the study begins.

public good A good or service that is jointly consumed by more than one person that is nonrival (cannot diminish the good to others when used) and nonexclusive (is available to everyone without exclusion).

qualitative analysis (or design) A fundamental research design that studies events or phenomenon of a non-numerical nature, typically of a behavioral or communication nature, and attempts to disclose underlying meanings and patterns of relationships.

quality-adjusted life-years A means of determining the value of life by adjusting for the quantity of life in years and the quality of life in status that occur as a result of an alternative, decision, intervention, or venture.

quantitative analysis (or design) A fundamental research design that studies events or phenomena of a numerical nature, typically through observations, interventions, precise measurements, and statistical probability predictions, to disclose underlying relationships of causality.

quasi-experimental design Quantitative research that is similar to experimental design, but without the advantage of randomization of subjects or interventions.

quick ratio A financial analysis tool (also known as an acid test) that is very effective in revealing an organization's liquidity.

receptivity testing Similar to concept testing in feasibility analysis, except an actual prototype product or limited service to a subpopulation of the targeted clientele is tested for its utility and acceptability.

regulatory impact analysis Cost-benefit analysis in government determination of regulatory policies and their impact on society.

resource sufficiency Adequacy of assets of an organization, not only in financial terms but also in access and availability of application.

resource sufficiency analysis An assessment of an organization intended to determine the adequacy of assets of an organization, not only in financial terms but also in access and availability of application.

retained earnings The accumulated amount of past and current earnings of an organization that are not disbursed (either maintained as a cash asset or invested into the organization).

retrospective longitudinal study An investigative study that examines data over time in a retrospective manner; often derived through the examination of documents and records.

retrospective research A form of longitudinal research that looks into the past for information and data collection; these studies are convenient as the data already exist, but somewhat less effective as the controls cannot be put into place before the study begins.

return on assets A financial analytical tool that reveals the relationship of an organization's earnings to its total assets as a measure of productivity or profitability; abbreviated ROA.

return on services A financial analytical tool for determining profitability by examining what percentage of revenue from services results in net income; known as return on sales in a production organization.

revenues The money earned by an organization through the delivery of services and other sources of income; an elemental aspect of the income statement.

root cause analysis A tool commonly used in continuous quality-improvement practices to illustrate contributing factors to a common problem and to aid in developing a solution.

scope of operations The capacity and breadth of an organization's operations in accordance with delivery models and practice standards.

scope of operations analysis An assessment of an organization intended to determine the capacity and breadth of an organization's operations in accordance with delivery models and practice standards.

secondary research question Research questions borne from the identified problem that modify or supplement the key research question; secondary research questions often seek additional information for clarification of the key research question.

selection bias A common threat of internal validity whereby choosing subject participation or exposing subjects to interventions is nonrandomized and often under some conscious or unconscious bias; this type of bias may influence outcomes.

self-reporting bias A type of internal validity threat that results from the subject providing information directly under the full awareness of the purpose; as it is human nature to depict oneself in the "best light," there may be some embellishment of data.

sensitivity analysis A step in cost-benefit analysis that attempts to measure the consequences of the impact categories of various alternatives and the effect each has on the others by acknowledging the presence of uncertainty.

shareholder's equity Found on the balance sheet, the recorded value of residual claims of all of the owners of the organization.

social discount rate The rate at which future benefits and costs should be discounted to reveal their present values.

statistical life The approximated value that an individual is willing to pay to avoid the risk of death; the economic equivalence of the social value of a human life.

status quo alternative In impact analysis, the problem solution alternative that does nothing, but keeps the situation the same; a means of comparative analysis by examining impact categories against the current situation.

straight-line depreciation A method of depreciation that is traditional and progressively depreciates the asset or good over the useful lifetime of the asset, less the recovery or end-of-life value; the depreciation is equivalent for each year depreciated.

subjective expected utility A theory that proposes that all decisions are subject to maximal utility of rational thought and all relevant factors are known.

sum-of-years depreciation A method of depreciation that places greater emphasis on the depreciation of an asset or good in

the earlier years of its useful lifetime by fractioning the depreciation in accordance with the number of useful years as a depreciation rate.

SWOT analysis A common strategic planning approach that examines the strengths, weaknesses, opportunities, and threats of an organization; often compared to a feasibility analysis; a component of operational feasibility that has its basis in strategic planning of an organization; it reveals the alignment potential of a new initiative or venture with the organization's mission, vision, and goals.

technical feasibility An analytical process as a component of feasibility analysis that assesses the functional ability of an organization to proceed with an initiative or venture; it examines the scope of performance and the organization's skill sets as applicable to the pursuit.

telephonic survey A method of conducting a survey through the means of contacting the respondent via telephone; the interviewer follows a predetermined script and records the interviewee's responses.

testing effects A threat to internal validity caused by subjects being tested repeatedly; also a form of threat that results from the subject being aware of the testing process (see Hawthorne effect).

time order A criterion for variable selection that specifies that the effects resulting from the variable of interest has an impact on the dependent variable, and, so, must precede the independent variable in time.

time value of money A financial concept that recognizes that money changes value over time (typically a reduction toward the future) and enables financial and economic analysts to value future amounts of money in present-day equivalencies.

total assets Found on the balance sheet, all of the assets of an organization, including the current assets, fixed assets less depreciation, and all other assets owned.

total costs An economic principle used in breakeven analysis that includes all variable and fixed costs of an organization.

trend study A form of longitudinal research whereby the study population possesses some characteristic of study interest, but otherwise lacks any commonality.

typology A systematic classification of varying forms of a subject, concept, or categories based on similar characteristics; a classification or categorization.

unit hour utilization analysis (UHUA) A performance measure adapted from the manufacturing industry for application to EMS that assesses efficiency of utilization of services per unit of time.

units of analysis An important element in study design that specifies the what or whom being studied.

value Not just the monetary equivalency of a product or service, but also the quality it brings to the organization.

variable costs The costs in an organization that are associated with operation and are subject to fluctuation in amounts coincident with the changes in volume of services.

variables A known or unknown element in an equation that is representative of a set of attributes unique to that element.

welfare economics A type of microeconomics that deals with equal distribution of income or goods or services to society as a whole to ensure well-being; the basis for Pareto efficiency.

working capital The amount of earned income that an organization has generated that is available for expenses, investments, and new acquisitions; derived by deducting current liabilities from current assets; also known as net current assets.

Index

www.ingramcontent.com/pod-product-compliance
Lightning Source LLC
Chambersburg PA
CBHW081526220326

41598CB00036B/6348